Bedtime Stories for Adults

26 Relaxing Sleep Stories to Help You Overcome Anxiety & Insomnia and Deep Sleep (Meditation & Self-Hypnosis)

Sandra Moreau

© Copyright 2020 - All rights reserved.

The content contained within this book may not be reproduced, duplicated or transmitted without direct written permission from the author or the publisher.

Under no circumstances will any blame or legal responsibility be held against the publisher, or author, for any damages, reparation, or monetary loss due to the information contained within this book, either directly or indirectly.

Legal Notice:

This book is copyright protected. It is only for personal use. You cannot amend, distribute, sell, use, quote or paraphrase any part, or the content within this book, without the consent of the author or publisher.

Disclaimer Notice:

Please note the information contained within this document is for educational and entertainment purposes only. All effort has been executed to present accurate, up to date, reliable, complete information. No warranties of any kind are declared or implied. Readers acknowledge that the author is not engaged in the rendering of legal, financial, medical or professional advice. The content within this book has been derived from various sources. Please consult a licensed professional before attempting any techniques outlined in this book.

By reading this document, the reader agrees that under no circumstances is the author responsible for any losses, direct or indirect, that are incurred as a result of the use of the information contained within this document, including, but not limited to, errors, omissions, or inaccuracies.

Table of Contents

1. In a Wonderful Desert 5

2. Drive to the Farm 20

3. The Party and Anthony 33

4. The Human Mind 40

5. Our Dreams 45

6. Cleanest Water..55

7. The Sweet Surrender 63

8. The Childhood Blanket..70

9. Floating Across a Pale Blue Sky......................................77

10. A Forty-something-year-old Woman 86

11. Hold the Key to Your Relief...90

12. The Amazing Princess 99

13. A Sense of Being out Bird Watching 102

14. The Adventurous Shark 111

15. Sitting at the Roulette Table 119

16. Travel to Greece 126

17. A Different Dive 137

18. A Strange Day 144

19. The Adult Friendship 152

20. At the Bar 175

21. An Incredible Trip 183

22. In the Favorite Diner 188

23. Trip to Barcelona 194

24. The Sleep Rainbow 208

25. The Famous Writer 214

26. On a Hot Air Balloon 220

1. In a Wonderful Desert

Jenny stuck her face out the window, letting the brisk night air roll over her, whipping her hair back.

The kids were asleep

The car was quiet, and the only sound in the night was the sound of the tires rolling sibilantly along the road.

Her husband drove so she could relax, and though sleep tugged at her eyelids, she wanted to stay awake a little longer.

They were headed out on vacation, which meant a drive across the desert, and she loved the desert. It was always so peaceful, and as a child, her parents had often taken them out in the RV into the desert to experience a little bit of camping outside of the usual spots.

The desert at night was one of the most incredibly beautiful places Jenny had known in her life.

A deep blue sky twinkling with stars blanketed the land, flat but for the buttes that occasionally rose up in the distance.

Cacti stood tall, their spiny arms raised, the moving shadows making them appear as if waving at the passing car.

Deep shadows pooled in the small ravines and gullies as they drove past.

Night birds gave their hooting cries, and the steady chirp of crickets made Jenny drowsy.

Her head nodded once, then twice. She yawned so hard that tears started in her eyes.

Jenny tried to shake away the sleepiness but her eyelids remained heavy.

Blinking through the fatigue, she thought that the full moon looked a little funny

Clouds had passed in front of its center, making it resemble a giant yellow number "8."

At last, she laid her head back against the seat and let the wind rushing through the open window soothe her.

She closed her eyes and soon her dreams wandered into the desert night.

Just like one of the stories in her book….

* * *

A young Jaina stepped out of the family camper and into the clear night.

The sky was a vast night blue canvas upon which trails of stars were painted.

A pale light loomed on the horizon as the sunset faded from the sky.

She loved the nights out here, camping where you could hear the coyotes and the crickets.

No sound of cars, no doors slamming, no machines rattling. Only the soft whoosh of the open air and the sounds of the creatures that lived in the desert.

Jaina liked to pretend she was one sometimes. She wondered what it would be like to live like the desert birds or the mice or even the snakes and lizards.

Jaina imagined a little kangaroo mouse, like the kind she had seen last night on the edge of the firelight. Her gaze wandered across the hundreds of little paths and hiding places visible in the light of the fire.

She knew better than to wander too far and disturb a sleeping stinger of some kind, but here, in the little ring of rocks and cacti where they had parked the camper, she was safe to explore.

Elsewhere, a mouse tentatively hopped out of its little burrow—to the mouse, it was a cave, but to the world outside, it was barely a hole. For a young kangaroo mouse, it was the only home she needed.

As the night fell dark and chilly upon the desert, she was on a mission: to simply enjoy the night. On other nights, she might seek out food, or friends, but tonight was more like a journey through the dreams of the desert itself.

She might have been a traveler, safely asleep in her den, or perhaps blessed enough to feel part of another dreamer's adventure.

When the lines between worlds blurred, story and reality were not so different, after all.

Tonight, she was safe to explore.

Her burrow opened out onto a dried-up riverbed. It had been many long months since water coursed down the channel, and it would not tonight, but the land itself remembered the taste.

The mouse did not need the water to survive. To her, it was a strange and wondrous occurrence when the skies opened up and poured cold drops upon the desert.

Then the waterways would run like torrents and she would have to hide in a nice, cozy, dry burrow.

Smooth rocks and dusty shrubs currently filled the riverbed. Deep shadows enshrouded them. A single cricket stood atop a nearby rock and belted out its high-pitched night song.

The mouse stopped and the looked at it.

"Beautiful night for music," said the mouse.

"Music is for every night!" said the cricket, and he stopped playing long enough to answer her.

"The night, she sings to me. Does she sing to you?"

"I only hear your song," said the mouse. "But I feel like there is more out there tonight, so I am going to find it."

"Then I wish you luck!" And the cricket began to play again, this time a song of exploration and discovery.

The hopeful tune accompanied the mouse as she bounded down the riverbed from perch to perch.

Tall rocks like cliffs overlooked the path, littered with dust and spotted with tough little shrubs and weeds.

The tracks of other nocturnal creatures also formed trails in the sun-baked terrain.

The mouse recognized many of them: snakes, lizards, desert tarantulas, and her own trails from past nights.

Each was a snapshot of life in the desert. To outsiders, the land seemed arid and barren, barely able to sustain life.

As the mouse journeyed through this very vibrant world, it was all very much alive with an entire world hidden in the stones and sand.

A constant cacophony of bird whistles filled the air, alternating like the creaking metal joints of a wheel.

Hidden just behind a line of rocks, some insect crawled with a sibilant scratch. It was a huge black beetle, gleaming in the night, its antlers on proud display as it thrust one of the rocks, bigger than its own body, aside to make a path.

"Oh. Good. Evening." The beetle spoke in a very slow and plodding monotone.

"You are very strong!" said the mouse, her own voice excited. She had never seen such a beetle before and found him endlessly fascinating.

"Oh. Maybe. I. Am." The beetle crawled slowly into the riverbed, now becoming a highway for the passage of the desert's many living creatures as the sunset faded and night deepened. "But. You.

Are. Very. Fast!" The beetle turned and began to crawl in the direction the mouse had come from.

"If you need a place to stay for the night, please use my burrow! I won't be back until the morning!"

The mouse wanted to be charitable. She had never seen anything like this beetle and was hoping to meet him again, but she could not stay. Adventure called!

"Thank. You." The beetle stopped and turned his great horned head. "Maybe. I. Will!"

"You are welcome!" The mouse squeaked with delight and bounded down the path again.

A bird sleeping in the arm of a cactus overlooking the path awoke as she paused and looked down at her.

It was a wren, brown, white, and fluffy, like the mouse. It waved its wings at her and then tucked its head into sleep again.

But the mouse felt fortunate. The wren's feathers reminded her of her family, and it made her all the more excited to see them again.

Many shapes loomed up out of the dark. The cacti were as towers, but in the shrubs, a warm wind rustled.

The mouse felt as though she ran into a forest, which moved endlessly as she turned a bend in the riverbed.

The banks were much higher here when in days past the river had rushed through with greater strength.

Long ago, the voice of those waters had filled the land, and all who came to this little valley would hear them.

For the song of the river was a timeless one, at once ancient and yet eternally young.

Always changing, but always retaining the same purpose in life.

The little mouse climbed the steep banks, hopping from purchase to purchase, until at last, she scrabbled up to the very top, to her a bluff overlooking a mighty riverbed.

There she saw the channel that the water had once delved into the land itself and she wondered what it must have been like, back when the desert's dreams were full of water.

As if in answer to her desire, a sudden rumbling in the earth accompanied a liquid roar.

The mouse looked up the slope of the riverbed and saw it coming, a torrent of silvery water that rolled forth with a clamor.

In the foam and spray as it came, shapes of the desert formed and then melted away just as quickly, each an embodiment of the lives that the river touched.

A great spider appeared upon a web of water droplets and then blended into a clutch of newly hatched snakes experiencing their first taste of the warming sun.

The curious snakes dove into the waves and up emerged owls with wings spread wide, and eyes like lamps.

The owls flapped their splashing wings and became bats, sending out a song that echoed through the water.

When the bats dropped back to the water out sprang hares and bighorn sheep, and behind them leaping deer and laughing foxes.

The river rushed past, and as it came, the very air shimmered and seemed to change.

A smell of ozone followed.

Thunder crackled in the sky far above.

Rain fell, eager to join the river on its course through the dusty flatlands.

All at once, as if awoken from slumber, countless voices rose in a murmur at the rain's sweet song.

This was one of the miracles of the desert, an occurrence so rare that the parched earth scarcely recalled the taste of water.

Now the little kangaroo mouse got to witness what it had always dreamed of—and it was truly beyond imagination.

One of the wrens landed on the outcropping beside her and shook its rain-soaked feathers.

"So lovely!" he said in a loud voice belying his little size, not much bigger than the mouse herself.

"What a night to be alive! It is said that often the desert dreams of the rain, but rarely do the dreams come true."

He turned to the mouse. "Good evening, friend! Do you come here to see the river, too?"

The mouse hopped excitedly up and down. "I wanted to see what this place was like when the great water was still here! And now I can! But is this real or are we seeing the past?"

The wren laughed in answer. "Friend that is the wrong question to ask!"

"What is the right question?" the little mouse said, eager to know the answers she sought. But the cagey old wren only laughed again.

"The question is not what is, or was, or what will be. The question is simply: what does this mean to now?"

Despite her best attempts, the young mouse simply could not understand. "What do you mean, Mr. Wren? I don't understand that, either!"

The bird lifted his wings and spread them wide. "Because you are young, and you seek out the purpose of the dream. You look for what course the river runs to understand it, but that is not the river's way. The river flows upon whatever course awaits it. The river does not question why it simply experiences the thrill of its adventure."

"Am I not to question, then?" The little mouse felt dejected, but soon the wren lifted her spirits again.

"You should always question! Always seek the truth behind the dream. What you must learn one day is that sometimes the dream is the truth itself, and the truth is the dream. Can one exist without the other? Do you feel the water, hear its voice, and bask in its embrace? Yes? Then the river is real, whatever its origin or path."

With that, the wren bid her goodnight and flew off into the rain, whistling loudly and cheerfully.

The little mouse clapped her paws and watched as the river rushed past, telling the story of the desert's history and foretelling its future.

Year by year, she returned to that spot to experience the same dream, and year by year, she grew to understand what the old wren had meant.

One day she became a mother and a grandmother and patriarch to a large and thriving mouse family, and still, she came back to that spot, long after the wren had gone.

One day, she stood there as the river crashed through, and another young mouse climbed up to that very same hill.

His little eyes grew wide as he observed the momentous event; overcome with the magic of the waters he had seldom known. And he asked the very same question that the little kangaroo mouse had once asked of the wren.

"I have never seen anything like this! Is this real?"

The old kangaroo mouse smiled.

* * *

Jaina awoke with a yawn. She had not even realized that she had fallen asleep until she felt the first few raindrops on her skin.

The fire had died down, but there was a curious little mouse standing near it.

Jaina smiled and started to reach out to it but the mouse hopped away...though not out of fear.

It jumped for the sheer joy of the desert night. As she watched it go, Jaina felt like she had known a little of what that was like.

Then a bird atop the camper called to her, a little brown wren before it flew off into the night as well.

Jaina watched it go as the rain began to fall drop by drop.

She heard the songs of the crickets and the cicadas, and in the distance, a coyote howled to greet the rain.

Even the fire, sizzling as it was with each drop, seemed to be sighing in relief at the welcome return of an old friend.

She looked up into the stars and breathed in the sweet smell of fresh rain, the tang of parched dust soaking up the moisture, and the cool caress of the breeze.

Long after Jaina went back inside the camper that night, she dreamed of dusty plains, rivers rushing, and mice hopping freely.

As the night passed and the sky began to lighten again, an old kangaroo mouse hopped into the campsite. She stared at the camper curiously for a long moment.

"I wonder what they are dreaming?" the mouse said to herself.

Then she had a strange feeling that she already knew, and the thought brought her peace. With the sun coming up, it was time for her to return to the burrow where food, slumber, and family awaited.

She hopped away, content in sharing her desert dreams with all the others in her blessed home.

As she neared her burrow, the old mouse heard the cry of a wren.

Then, in the distance, she thought she heard the whoosh and burble of rushing waters.

She smiled and closed the door to listen to the water while she slept.

Water Gazing

Sitting and watching the river flow

Wondering where it is that it will go

Never to tarry at the same place

Always a forward-moving race

I cast my troubles and cares to the river

I watch the eddies and currents until I shiver

Water, it washes all my strife away

And to it, I return to play

Desert Night

The heat of the day has gone at last

And the cool midnight blankets this land, so vast

Some might see this panorama as desolate and bare

But if you look, life is thriving everywhere

The coyote howls in the distance of the night

Under a desert sky, no moon but stars are bright

A mouse scurries from his home, in search of a meal

Avoiding the night predators, he has nerves of steel

In a saguaro cactus silhouetted in the dark

Is the hidden home, of a sleeping little lark

An owl hoots somewhere up in the blackened skies

Searching for the prey that will not escape his sharp eyes

The desert night has a multitude of surprises to behold

It can only be witnessed by those who are bold

Look closely and it's secrets it shall reveal

The desert night, such mysterious appeal

Sunrise on the Horizon

The sun wakes up from his slumber and begins his accent

As the moon maiden finishes her early morning decent

The sunrise on the horizon in a magnificent sight

First, pinks and then oranges and then the yellow so bright

Sunrise over the ocean, one of nature's treasures

Watching it every morning is one of life's simple pleasures

The earth warms under his nurturing rays

Waves reflect his light back in awesome displays

Sunrise it the most perfect time of day

Everything is fresh and new and ready for work or play.

Nothing is better than basking in the light of the newly born sun

When the day has just begun

Desert Skies

Into the desert night, we walk, hand in hand

Gently we place a blanket upon the sand

Cacti dot the landscape making up nature's skyline

Here in the desert, barrenness and life combine

Millions of stars are close enough to touch

We spot the big dipper, and Orion and such

A shooting start tears a path of light

And I make a wish that we could live forever in this night

I am surprised by the unexpected chill in the air

The daytime had been so hot, I must compare

Suddenly another meteor makes its way to the ground

And soon falling stars are all around

The desert sky is a magical sight to behold

I know we will still come to watch, even when we have grown old

Here we are surrounded by the beautiful rugged charm

Then with the sunrise, we leave arm in arm.

The Moon

I see the moon rising above the mountain top

The night sky is illuminated with her magic

Clouds drift slowly by, but her light will not stop

Higher she travels in the sky

Watching everyone from her vantage point

As the long, lovely night passes by

Lady Luna shine your moonbeams down

Fill my soul with laughter

And spread happiness and peace throughout the town

Now I watch as the moon sets into the sea

Gone to bed for the day

But I smile knowing that tonight she will return to me.

2. Drive to the Farm

Jenny needed the drive to clear her head.

It had been a long week. Her boss was breathing down her neck and at home, Kirsty was competing for attention with a nine-month-old baby.

Her husband was also working long hours and often out of town, leaving Jenny to handle the kids, coordinate the bills, and do all the chores.

Sometimes she just felt like her neck was so tense she could barely turn her head.

Always another unexpected issue to pop up, always something going wrong.

That was life, she told herself, but it did not make it any easier when she was up all night fretting over a looming bill or an appointment.

These drives out in the summer afternoon were a wonderful way to clear her head.

She would call her sister and have Aunt Julia come and watch the kids while she sometimes went out for a few hours just to think.

On the other hand, she would even bring Kirsty and the baby with her, out to the old country roads outside the city.

Sometimes she would even drive back as far as the farms where she used to go and visit her grandparents, even staying whole summers out there.

Helping to till the fields, plant the crops, or feeding the animals (which was always her favorite). And the nights!

Listening to the steady voice of a distant creek, and the soft roar of wide-open spaces.

The occasional bleating of an animal or the long, mournful-sounding cries of the peacocks. A rush of feathers as a bird flew overhead, returning to its nest to sleep.

The playful thumps of the barnyard cats coming indoors for a meal and to chase one another.

A wide expanse of grass and golden hills opened up before her, slowly drifting past.

The road dipped and rose again, winding its slow way out through the countryside.

Sprawling patches of tilled fields and growing wheat gave way to beautiful farmhouses and old, weathered barns in the distance.

She wondered what it would be like to live in such a place, enjoying the fresh air and the night skies full of stars.

Her grandparents had so often said it was the single best thing they had ever done, making the move out to the country.

While Jenny loved her life, its many challenges made her long for something simpler.

The afternoon grew warmer. White puffs of cloud lazily floated through a cerulean sky.

Jenny found her mind wandering back to some of her favorite days as she drove through a corridor of tall trees on either side.

A little excitement built in her belly, just like it did when she was a child, because on the right side of the road ahead, the treeline thinned out and then stopped, and as soon as it did one could see her grandparents' farm down at the end of a very long gravel driveway.

Every time she drove down this way, her heart did a little leap as she approached that last tree lining the road.

There it was! A small white patch glimpsed in the distance, across wide fields, standing amid other buildings: an old barn, the ruins of an old house now used for the chickens (and the cats), a hay shack, pens for the pigs, cows, and horses.

She saw the cows in the field, though they looked like small black and white lumps from this distance.

It had been a few months since she had visited Grandma Belinda and she decided now was as good a time as any.

Grandpa Dale had passed a few years back but had his ashes mixed with the soil of the farm fields.

He always wanted to be a part of the growth and lives of that place he loved so much, and even as she turned down the long driveway, she saw he felt his warm smile beaming upon her like the afternoon sun.

The gravel crackled beneath the car tires.

Long before she would ever get close to the house, the dogs' ears would perk up and they would go running and barking home—or out to meet her once they recognized the car.

There they came now, barking excitedly as they rushed across the field to meet her, while she had to take the driveway around the long bend and finally past the older buildings to the farmhouse itself.

Jenny rolled down the window and smiled as the dogs kept pace with her car, barking their greeting.

"Hey there! Did you miss me, guys? Go and tell Grandma that I'm here!"

And as if they had understood, the dogs did turn and ran back for the house, but Belinda needed no warning.

There she was standing in front of the house, now walking out to meet Jenny as she drove up.

Grandma had a layer of dirt and grime on her clothes; she had already been out that day working somewhere on the farm.

The woman was a marvel in her ability to keep going, even despite her age when Jenny felt like she could barely muster the energy to get through her own challenges.

"Grandma!" Jenny was quick to greet her grandmother with a hug.

Belinda smiled as she embraced her granddaughter.

"It's good to see you, dear. I have been thinking about you lately, you know. I was hoping you'd come to visit soon!"

Jenny then knelt and played with the dogs, one a rambunctious Border Collie, the other a mutt with the most joyous wagging tail any dog had ever known.

They flopped and rolled on the lawn before her, so excited they could barely contain themselves long enough to be petted.

Jenny laughed, and as she did so, weeks of worry and stress that had built lines upon her features smoothed away, weight lifted from her shoulders, none of it ever to return.

The sheer joy of being out here, in the warmth and sun, while the entire mountain around them bloomed, overcame any hardships.

Deep shades of green filled all of her sights, as the mountain rose still further up in the distance, and a steep incline led down to a little creek valley behind the house.

The forest was at its height of growth in the fullness of its Summer.

The smells of fresh water mingled with the scents of evergreen, the heady aroma of wheat, even the unpleasant animal pen smells were tied to memories.

The whole experience was a life unto itself, a story that unfolded anew each day with the crowing of the roosters to green the dawn.

A peacock sounded off in the tree above the old house that had been converted into a chicken coop. Several others also howled in response.

Jenny loved that sound now, but when she was a kid, she thought it sounded like they were saying, "Help! Help!"

A light breeze stirred her hair and gently rumbled in her ears.

She took in a deep breath through her nose and let out a long and satisfied sigh.

"Grandma, it's so good to see you. I went for a drive and I just ended up here. I thought I'd see how you were doing."

Belinda smiled. "I was just about to go and give the animals their dinner. Do you want to help?"

"Do I?" Jenny's eye lit up.

Feeding the animals was always her favorite part as a kid. Grandma knew that.

She nodded toward the animal pens. "Come on. I already knew the answer to the question."

The dogs followed the women as they walked around the farmhouse toward the pens.

Grandma asked Jenny about her life, and Jenny told her how things were going.

She tried to make it sound like everything was fine, but Grandma had keener ears and eyes than that.

"I know you're stressed, sweetheart, but trust me: you're doing well. You've got a great family and you're making it work."

"I just feel like it's so much of a struggle sometimes, you know, Grandma? Is it normal to feel this way? Like you don't have it under control?"

Belinda chuckled.

"Yes, honey, it is. In fact, I would be more worried if you said you did not even have to worry. However, you are doing what you should be doing. Raising a family on your own isn't easy, but it's also the most beautiful challenge you'll ever experience."

She opened up the weather-beaten door of a large shack, and the smell of animal feed drifted into the air.

"You just have to remember that no one controls it all. It is okay that you cannot do anything. And it's okay to take some time away to get a new perspective."

Belinda handed Jenny a large metal cup, which Jenny gladly scooped into the animal feed.

Dust swirled upward as she brought the now-heavy cup up full of feed pellets.

She followed her grandmother out to the pigpens and poured the feed into the troughs, and then back to the shack to do it again.

The horses and cows also received multiple cups of the feed, but then Jenny and her grandmother-retrieved armfuls of hay from the shack and tossed them over the fences for the bigger animals.

Soon all were crunching happily at their food.

One of the horses, a big mottled silver and white horse named Bingo, came to the fence.

Jenny had named him in her creative youth, shrilly singing the song as she did so, of course, but he had always been a favorite of hers.

She gently patted the horse's forehead and snout, and he thanked her with a thunderous snort.

Bingo went back to the food, while Jenny returned to her grandmother.

They walked along a trail past the house and down to the converted coop.

Rusted tractors derelict for many years sat in the tall grasses, and other things like mossy, decayed wooden fences added the weight of history to the trail.

The sun began to sink a little, disappearing over the forested mountain, casting its light but not beating down upon them.

The air-cooled and carried with it a sense of freshness and vitality.

Jenny thought she could breathe in that air forever.

"You know, you're a lot stronger than you think, Jen."

Belinda looked over at her granddaughter as they walked.

"You realize that you've been smiling this whole time? Just like when you were a girl. Same lopsided grin and everything."

"Aw, Grandma."

"It's okay to feel overwhelmed or frustrated, dear. However, the important part is this. What you are doing right now. Taking some time to let it all go. To reconnect."

"I wish I could live out here all the time. I do love the city, but this is so much more relaxing."

Belinda looked around, her gaze sweeping across the entire plot of land.

"It is nice, dear, but its work, no matter how you look at it. That is what we do. We take care of our families until they don't need us anymore…."

But Grandma smirked as she turned back to Jenny, who grinned wide.

"But they always need us!"

"Exactly."

Their footsteps thumped on the floor of the old house as they walked in to feed the chickens.

A heat lamp shone over the nesting box where the chicks chirped.

One wall in the front room held shelves of boxes for the hens to lay their eggs, and branch-like perches in front of them.

Straw and feathers covered the floor.

Jenny loved the sounds the chickens made; the constant soft clucks and squawks had always been very relaxing to her.

The women spread the chicken feed on the ground just outside the door, and some in the hen room.

Most of the chickens gathered around them and followed them outside, recognizing their feeding time.

Jenny crouched down and reached out slowly to pet some of the chickens that came close.

They were docile and friendly creatures, and some of them looked at her before moving on to their food.

Jenny closed her eyes and listened to the sound: the scratching of their beaks on the ground, the soft flutter of their feathers, their clucks telling each other of the food they found. Peaceful. Simple.

Grandma's hand rested upon her shoulder.

"Even this, my dear Jen, should remind you. The chickens do what we do. Even now, they are calling to the others, telling their young of the food they have found. They are taking care of each other. Because that is a hen's job, dear. Our jobs are never finished! You just have to take that time to appreciate all the simple things, and be appreciated."

She held out a hand to help her granddaughter up.

"Come on. Let me make you dinner. It is our turn to eat. Then you can drive back and sleep a little more easily tonight."

Jenny took the proffered hand and they walked together back to the house.

Grandma cooked up a lovely dinner, and they shared stories, laughed over old memories, and Belinda gave her a parting gift.

"This horseshoe was the very first one I ever put on a horse. I did not know what I was doing. I was young like you, scared; worried I was not doing anything right. And you know what? All these years later, I kept this because of it as a reminder that I did get through it. That I was stronger than I thought. Now I want you to have it. And I want you to remind yourself every time you feel like you are not good enough that you are. You can get through it, too."

Jenny accepted the gift with tears in her eyes.

She thanked her grandmother many times.

The two of them shared a long and reluctant goodbye after dinner, and although Jenny hated to leave, as the sunlight receded from a clear sky and the fresh air rolled in through her window, she drove home with a lighter heart.

The road was empty but for Jenny and her dreams of a better life.

Dreams that she was working every day to foster, just like the chickens, just like her grandmother did.

The night was pleasantly cool and welcoming as she drove, settling like a blanket upon the fields and the forests.

She checked on the girls. Julia had fallen asleep while reading Kirsty a bedtime story, and the baby was asleep in her crib.

Jenny gently caressed the baby's cheek, then turned out the light and went to turn the lights out.

The house settled into the quiet hum of the peaceful summer nights.

Jenny paused to listen and had the feeling that her grandmother even now was doing the same thing.

When she laid down in her bed that night, Jenny dreamed of chickens and peacocks, riding over the open fields beside a stream that softly murmured to her with her grandmother's reassurances.

Summer night sounds drifted in through the window, along with the distant whinnying of a horse.

Fire Dancers

I see the dancers in the fire

In the flames, spiraling higher.

Spinning to their cracking song

Fire dancers, my mind dances along.

Fire dancers, burning all the night

Smoldering to slumber in the first morning light

For my forgotten frivolity, they make me yearn

Beautiful fire fae, will you return?

Frogs and Pollywogs

When I was a child, I found such delight

In frogs and pollywogs

When I would go down to the pond to play

I would forget my games and watch them all-day

How does this little swimmy, fishy thing

Become a creature that can jump and sing?

So much time I spent in contemplation

And my days I spent in anticipation

Now my days are filled with adult responsibility

That I have forgotten all about possibility

When and how it is not clear

But somehow the magic, it did disappear.

I think today I shall run away

And go back to the pond where I used to play

I sit on the wet, mossy logs

And spend the day watching frogs and pollywogs.

Summer at the Farm

I want to go back, for one more summer on the farm

And spend my afternoons on the front porch shelling peas

I will drink sweet tea and gossip with grandma and Aunt Louise

I will go out and hoe weeds from the garden

And pick green tomatoes to fry in a cast iron pan

The tomatoes will be lined up on the counter ready to can

Grampa will be out in the field on his tractor

Cutting down, and then bailing up the hay

All to ensure his cows have food some snowy winter day

When the sun goes down, Grandma will ring the dinner bell

And later we will sit on the porch and watch the fireflies

And then we shall retire, only to wake with the sunrise

If only, I could have one more summer on the farm

But all I have now are the sweet golden memories

That comes to my thoughts as gently as a summer breeze

3. The Party and Anthony

Anthony was a juggler in every sense of the word. He was so good at biting off more than he could chew, and somehow making it through whatever situation he had gotten himself into. When he was just a young boy, he put a lot of time and effort into teaching himself to be a literal juggler. He could remember nights were he and his father would practice in his backyard. His father would throw him a new ball, just as he was finding his stride with what he was already juggling.

He was a charismatic and funny young man and a shoo-in for the Circus. He relied a lot on his wit to carry him through life, which was something that he was loved for. He could walk into a sad room and have everyone on the floor laughing within minutes. Humor was a gift that ran in his family. He was a tall and lanky young man with a mess of dark hair atop his head. He used his slightly alien looks to his advantage because his arms were just the appropriate length to save him from being whacked in the face by any given object that he was juggling.

Anthony was always taking on new projects in an effort to keep boredom at bay. The young man would have done well to learn when to slow down and just enjoy a nice day off, but those were vulgar words to Anthony. He needed to always be busy. He would involve himself in marketing and event coordination for the circus. He enjoyed life on the road and wanted to see as much of everywhere as he possibly could. So, whenever the circus stopped in a new town, Anthony would be the first to go and hand out fliers and meet fans.

He was also quite involved in the social aspects of his job. Anthony loved getting to know people in the audience. He had a close relationship with all the other performers. He would make an effort to the best friend that he knew how to be. When someone was sad or needed a shoulder to cry on, they would call Anthony.

He was also a very talented performer and practiced his routines every single day.

It was not enough for him to just be the juggler, he also wanted to reach out and gain new skills. He tried his hand at balancing and then eventually

jugging fire rods. Anthony was a very ambitious young man and had a tendency to spread himself a little thin. He needed to keep many projects going at one time, including his daily practice.

The audience always cheered for Anthony though and his efforts always seemed to work out regarding learning new tricks. With his charm and wit, he was a crowd favorite at the Circus. People stood up in their seats after seeing him take on an impossible juggling feat. The crowds went wild from the moment he walked into the ring, until the moment that he took his bow and exited the stage. Anthony loved his job and thrived on the appreciation and adoration of others.

A rumor had been going around the circus one day, that next week would be Rachel's birthday. Rachel was a contortionist who Anthony was particularly fond of and the two had often spent time teaching one another new tricks. He immediately felt the urge to offer to plan her birthday party. He knew himself well enough to know that he already had a lot going on and he didn't need to take party planning on as a project too. At first, he managed to keep his mouth closed and just ignored all conversations about her birthday. This didn't last forever though, because his friendly nature got the better of him. Anthony eventually spoke up and offered to oversee the planning of a party in Rachel's honor.

The circus management was thrilled to hear this because he was successful with every project he took on. They offered to cover money for any materials he might need and wished him luck. The young man sighed; he knew that he had potentially made a mistake. Rachel was just such a good friend to him, and he could not stand the thought of someone else botching a very important birthday celebration. After all, his specialty was juggling.

The whole party was meant to be a surprise for Rachel, so there is no way that he could let on that he was planning such a grand celebration. This led to a lot of running around on Anthony's end though, as he had underestimated the amount of coordination that it took to put together a celebration of this magnitude.

He spent days and days rushing from practice to the store to buy all the supplies needed to outfit a party. He was also trying to learn a new routine in the process, which stretched his concentration out even more. He had a vision of the way that her birthday should be set up.

He wanted to use the big top and outfit it with a collection of folding tables, positioned end-to-end. Anthony also wanted to cover the whole area in streamers and banners. He needed balloons and a buffet and a nice place for the gifts to be stacked. All of these realizations were taking a toll on Anthony's ability to sleep and his attention to his own routine.

Anthony lay in bed awake at night creating a mental checklist of all of the supplies that he was going to need. He found himself becoming more and more stressed out by the idea of getting all of this done in less than a week. He had always been a strong believer in meditation. He sat up in bed and did his best to quiet his mind. Anthony was still getting the occasional rouge thought, but he would just let it pass. He only paid attention to his breath, and eventually, this was enough to allow him to achieve some rest.

The next day at practice, he was consistently dropping every pin he tried to juggle. He was having such a difficult time not letting his thoughts run away

during the session. One of his best friends noticed that Anthony looked worn out. Bruce (the resident strong-man) asked Anthony what was on his mind. He was hesitant to share his troubles at first, but he eventually gave up and told his friend about the party. Bruce looked shocked that he had not heard anything about this before. He offered to help Anthony with the food and said that he should ask everyone else to pitch in too.

This concept was completely foreign to Anthony, who was used to taking on the responsibility himself. He thanked his friend profusely for his offer and marked food off of his mental checklist. After some deliberation, he decided that Bruce was right, and he should enlist the help of others. This was a manifestation of his desperation because he prided himself on being self- sufficient.

Anthony began asking around the circus and found so many friends that were willing to help him with the task. He had always been there for everyone else when they needed him. He was now finding out how much his kindness meant to everyone else. He was overwhelmed with the amount of assistance he was being offered.

In that coming week, Anthony spent all of his time providing instructions to the others as to what tasks they could help him complete. Before he knew it, they had planned a celebration that was far more grand than anything that he had in mind initially. They all worked together in secret. Each of the performers was functioning in tandem with the others, working like the cogs inside of a watch.

Bruce had planned a stunning menu, with all of Rachel's favorite foods.

Anthony had instructed him to make her favorite cake. She loved white cake with buttercream frosting and candy pieces in and on top. Bruce was a master at decorating cakes and ended up with something that could have come directly out of a princess's dream.

The animal performers worked together to come up with an activity that they could show off for Rachel, in her honor. The lion was an especially good friend of Rachel and he was excited to learn how to do a flip, in an effort to surprise her. She had always commented that she would pay to see him incorporate gymnastics into his show.

The clown and the trainers worked together to perfect the decorations, with Ellen the elephant helping in this area too. They all enjoyed the art of design and were happy to assist Anthony in making Rachel's party so special. Everyone was having so much fun working together, that Rachel's birthday was accidentally becoming their most celebrated occasion in the year. The young acrobat had even offered to lead everyone in singing 'Happy Birthday', as she had the voice of an angel. A young apprentice to the ringleader would trick Rachel into entering the big top, where she would then find the surprise of a lifetime.

On the night of the party, no one was able to find the birthday girl. Anthony found himself getting more and more nervous. If she were to walk in before everything was ready, then it would feel like all this effort was for naught. He wanted so badly for the night to go off smoothly. The young ringleader was just wandering around aimlessly, trying to find their guest of honor.

The finally finished setting up all the decorations, and the food was ready.

Anthony had also received word that Rachel was in her trailer alone. The ringleader had mentioned that she was crying and refused to leave her trailer with him because she was not having a good day. Anthony told him to take over the direction of everyone and he set off on his own to find Rachel.

Anthony knocked on her trailer and a teary-eyed Rachel answered the door. He asked what was wrong and she told him that she was upset that her parents could not be here with her today. This was the first birthday that she has ever celebrated on the road, and she just felt like she didn't mean much to anyone. Anthony convinced the young lady to leave her trailer and take a walk with him. This was not difficult for him, because everyone came to Anthony when they were sad. The juggler told her jokes and tried to improve her mood, all while steering their path in the direction of the big top.

Rachel was so upset that she didn't even notice that Anthony was clearly directing them toward the tent. The inside of the big top was dark, as everyone was hiding and waiting for the birthday girl to arrive. She gave Anthony a sideways look as he held a flap to the dark tent open and ushered her inside.

The moment that the pair were inside, the staff, management, and other performers all jumped out and yelled "SURPRISE!". Rachel began crying tears of joy as she realized that she was important. She was taken aback by all of the planning and effort that went into her party. Tears streaked her smiling face as she hugged her friend.

As the festivities ramped up that evening, the performers could be heard laughing from far outside the tent. Anthony felt such a sense of unity among his

circus family. They had all come together to do such a lovely thing. He was so proud. He was also astounded that all he had to do was ask for help, and it was given freely. That night was something that Rachel would remember forever. Just when she felt like the world had forgotten her, her friends made her birthday the largest event of the year.

4. The Human Mind

Tonight, we are going to witness the power of the human mind. An extraordinary existence that lies within you and the power within it has so much untapped potential. We are going to tap into that genius potential to give you the most relaxing and serene peace that your body and mind have ever experienced. First, you must clear your mind. Let's do this with an organizational approach. Imagine a room; it can be stark white, it can be an ordinary office; maybe it's a storage room, or an extraterrestrial room that is dark with sleek modern touches. This room will be your way to file and organize your thoughts, putting them away for the night.

Let us start collecting those thoughts, by exploring your thought super highway and gathering everything we can find. Collect the thoughts however you need; if they are organized maybe you can set up a road block. Position yourself to slow, then halt the thoughts, processing which way they need to go. Compressing the thoughts into tiny manageable pieces. Maybe your thoughts are scattered, you can lay a net or a trap, and gather them all up at once? Then take each thought, figure out what it is, assign it to a file. As all the thoughts ramble and bounce around in your mind, stop them and gather them into a pile. Maybe some thoughts are linked together, place them within the same file or box; however big you need that storage bin or containment system to be. Your stack is growing higher and higher as all the thoughts from the day leave your thought highway and go into your manageable file system.

Once you have a hefty pile, you lift it up. The weight feeling like a burden and weighing you down, you take the thoughts to your organizational room. Let's begin filing away these thoughts.

Stacking them, filing them, whatever you need to do to clean up your mind space. Making things nice, tidy, and neat. Take your time, go through every thought, making sure it is tucked away, not going to fall off and ramble its way back onto the thought highway. If you feel any loose thoughts escaping, making their way back onto the thought highway, let it go, don't fight it. Finish putting away what you have now, these thoughts are ready to be put to rest. Once everything is put in its place, go back to the highway for a last sweep. Any errant thoughts can be grabbed up now. Catch those thoughts and take them back to the organization room. Are all your thoughts tucked away? If yes, your mind is blank and ready to explore? If no, take a moment and keep collecting and storing until you're ready to move on.

You leave the organization room behind you now. You travel through your mind, we're going to tap into the parts you do not use often enough. You can visualize your brain, the parts you use often are alive and electric. As you pass these parts by, allow them to calm down. Let them rest, they have done enough for today, we don't need them for what we are going to do. You pass by the central part, the one that controls your breathing, you heart rate, gently caress it. Let it know it can relax too, it can slow down. Feel your breathing calm, your heart rate a soft cadence; the reassurance that life is within you and will continue to be so in the morning. As you feel your mind relaxing you continue to travel through. Passing the parts, you do not use enough, seeing them with their soft warm glow, welcoming you to tap into them. Once you have located the untapped potential, touch it. Reach up your arms and stretch them long. Stretch your torso and back, twist to reach it. Make your legs long all the way to your toes. Now you feel it, you're touching this dull area and a warm sensation is starting to come alive and you can feel it washing over you. It starts to warm up and emit a little happy glow that travels all through your body. Your muscles start to relax as the warmness caress it, your mind feels pleasant, bubbling and cloudy, until it sinks into the warm, soft light, then you can see a vivid green field all around you.

The sky is blue, the tall grass, soft and green. Your entire body feels warm and relaxed. Let's see if this is the true potential of your mind with a little test. Imagine yellow dandelions growing all over the field. Big ones, small ones. Count them as you add the yellow dandelions, until you can't count. There's too many, millions and millions of yellow flowers surrounding you with happiness and joy. This is the power of your mind, if your mind isn't cooperating then you're not ready for this area. Don't give up, go back, explore your brain, find another untapped area and keep trying. You will find one that will let you explore. Once you're in a warm area and you see the field that you can control, you are there. Now that we are all there let's practice this new and pleasing sensation of control, turn the dandelions into to their fluffy white flowers, ready to release their seeds into the world. All around you, in a field full of white fluffy dandelions. Pick one up. Take a deep breath in, then blow it out slowly. Watching the seeds spiral from the flower into the air. As the seeds float back to the earth, steady yourself. This is just a very small power that rests inside you, it can do so much more. Take another deep breath in as you pick another dandelion. Exhale as you blow those seeds and come to terms with the fact you are a genius. You are capable of anything you set your mind to. Rest and relaxation can help you tap into that genius.

You command your mind and body. Right now, you command them to relax. Your entire body is soft, relaxed, and pliable. Your mind is warm, enriched, and welcoming to the thoughts of your tapped genius potential. You can go anywhere in the world right now, without leaving this state of relaxation. Where do you want to go? Picture that place; is it an ocean shore, a busy city, a small village, or a place you know well? What does it smell like? What can you hear? What can you see? How does it make you feel? Take a moment and enjoy this place, explore the sensations. Is it everything you hoped it would be?

This is your mind allowing you to experience the most wonderful sensations whenever you want it to. This power is incredible. You want to be on a beach in Greece, done. You want to be in the mountains in Asia, done. You want to be anywhere in space or time, you can do that. You are a wonderful, amazing creature, with limitless abilities as you bring yourself into ultimate relaxation at the same time. Would you like to see what else your mind is capable of?

Picture the tallest building in the world. Now get to the top of it. How does your mind get you there? Do you instantly appear on the top of the building? Do you walk up to the building, enter, and take an elevator? Do you start the arduous task of climbing the stairs? Do you gear up and climb the side of the building? Or maybe you come from above, using a parachute as you fall from a plane to land on top of the tallest building in the world. So many possibilities can spring from one simple suggestion. If you can get to the top of this building, then you can do anything. Take your time, or get it done quickly. It doesn't matter, because all the potential to do it, is inside your mind.

Can you understand now how beautiful and creative your mind is? Your mind can grow and continue to astound you every day, if you let it. Listen to your mind, let it guide you... Let your mind connect with your heart, picture the direct link between the two. This connection will know what you want the most in this life. Do not stop it, do not slow it down. Let it carry you away, showing you your hopes and dreams and how you can achieve them. Stay in this state of relaxation, do not let the errant thoughts break out of their storage room. They are locked away, stored nice and neatly for tomorrow. Tonight, is not about any of those thoughts, quickly lock that door, then forget it. It is about you, who you are, what you want, and how you are going to get it.

Everything becomes clear and easy to manage. Just like organizing your thoughts, your mind can control and process anything you bring its way. Let it take over, just as it took you into this deep relaxation. Once you are in total control of your mind, then you can shut it down and go to sleep. Enjoy your peaceful rest, and I look forward to seeing your genius potential in the world.

5. Our Dreams

Almost all of us have had a dream that we are flying.

Sometimes you have wings.

Sometimes you are just gliding through the air like a superhero.

Often times, when we take flight in our dreams, it is symbolic of freedom and a way for us to become connected to letting go of our fears about life in general.

Flying has been described in the legends of old myths and folktales describing a flying person as having special powers.

These tales will always lead you to a form of self-discovery in which you take control of your journey, your destiny.

You are the captain and you know exactly where to fly, how high, and when to land.

Planting your feet on the solid ground all day can be hard, especially if you have a challenging or difficult situation or people in your life, or if you have a hard time processing your feelings and emotions.

Guided meditations and creative visualization are a huge part of how many enlightened people find their way to wholeness.

Your inner journey is just as valuable, meaningful, and important as your inner one.

When you follow your journey forward and trust yourself to fly in the right direction for yourself, then the stresses of life naturally fall away, and you can find peace, harmony, and balance with your whole life. So take a moment to connect with this positive notion.

Find your comfort zone, and let yourself fall into freely.

You are here to enjoy your life journey, not stress out about it all of the time.

You are here to have a purpose that is meaningful to you, not worry about whether or not you are doing a good enough job, or if you are successful enough.

You have always been and always are enough, and when you acknowledge that truth... that's when you can really fly.

Find your most comfortable position.

Find the parts of your body that feel restless or tense and shake them out.

Shake out any part of your body that has felt motionless for far too long.

Shake off anything that you might have absorbed from another person today, or from a challenging experience.

Shake off all of the drama that finds you when you are trying to find your peace of mind...

Inhale deeply and enjoy the way it feels to have control over your breath.

Exhale slowly and appreciate the way it feels to let go of something physically from your body.

Inhale slowly again, rejoicing in the fresh air that fills you up.

Exhale slowly and feel gratitude that you have come to this place of self-healing, to totally bond with your own creative inspiration and thoughts, to become even more closely connected to your inner self, free of drama, free of critique...no judgments.

Your breath has helped your body feel more relaxed.

You are sinking more deeply into your comfort and relaxation.

You are finding it easier to breathe naturally and smoothly.

You are feeling content just to be present here, taking good care of yourself, giving yourself all of the love, attention, and devotion that you need right now...

There are no rules on your inner journey.

All you have to do is appreciate your creative ability to see more clearly from your inner world.

How would you like to feel right now?

Do you feel the way you look in your reflection within your mind?

Do you look the way that you hope to feel?

As you gaze at your inner reflection, show yourself how you want to appear to yourself.

Give yourself the costume or uniform, the style or outfit that best suits how you want to feel within tonight.

You can change your hairstyle.

You can wear something you would normally never choose to put on in public.

Take a few moments as you breathe to appreciate the world you know in your mind.

You can be all of yourself here.

Allow yourself to appear the way you would like to feel right now...

You are going to feel like this for the rest of your guided meditation.

This is your world, and you can look and dress; however, you see fit.

You can change your outfit anytime you want to.

You can become whatever you really are deep down inside.

You might become an animal or a tree.

You might become a warrior or a princess.

You might become something that this world has never know before.

Enjoy the work of dressing yourself to fly.

When you are ready, inhale deeply...hold the breath for a count of three...and steadily release the breath from your body...

You are climbing up a staircase now.

It is made of stone, and it is carved as a spiral, going higher and higher.

It looks like the stairs within an ancient castle.

The castle is a part of your subconscious mind.

It is a place you can come to any time you need to dress yourself the way you want to or hope to feel inside and out...

The stairs are taking you up to the top of the castle.

When you get to the rooftop, you are able to walk out onto it.

The castle overlooks a great and vast kingdom.

It is familiar to you.

You have traveled here before.

As you look out over the land, you can point out to yourself other places you have already been: in a meadow, in a forest, by the ocean on a ship, in the clouds, by a river, in a garden of wonders...

This place holds the secret truth of you and your inner journey.

The landscape is wholly yours, and you can be anything here and do anything you want to help yourself find your truth and purpose.

It is where you will return as you quest for deeper meaning in your life, as you seek to know who you really are, deep down inside...

Standing on the castle roof, taking in the inner world of your mind, you are now able to take a new journey.

Your inner wisdom is what can help you find what you need to see right now, to help you relax and find peace of mind and inner calm.

You can let yourself find the right path when you trust yourself that you already know the answers.

You already know how to solve all of your problems and you can find it all right here in this inner kingdom of your body, mind, heart, and soul...

To take flight, all you have to do is face the world you have created in your thoughts and mind.

Take a moment to breathe and relax into this visual journey.

Take a moment to connect with your breath again and let yourself feel that moment before you take flight...

Stepping closer to the roof's edge, imagine you are outstretching your arms like they are wings, stretching far out to either side of you.

Underneath you are just castle grounds...or is it a waterfall that leads through a great misty fog that goes to another place in your kingdom?

When you look down, you see not the grounds of a castle, but a portal into another place and you can fly there, just by leaping off the rooftop and finding your flight.

The waterfall drops off into another place you cannot see.

It is where you can begin to teach yourself how to journey within your mind.

You can imagine anything you want...anything at all.

You can see beyond the reality of Earth and look at your inner universe with creativity and imagination.

You can picture a rainbow bridge to fly over that will lead you to another part of your kingdom.

You can picture a flying Pegasus who will transport you wherever you want to go.

Here, in your kingdom, there are no rules.

You are the one who decides how your world will look and how you will find your way forward...

Enjoy flying over your inner kingdom, and let keep unfolding for you.

Breathe steadily.

You can land anywhere you want and take off anywhere you want.

You are flying in order to get a bigger picture, greater scope and nothing is too big or too small here.

It is everything you ask it to be.

[give plenty of time for creative visualization and meditation here]

Your world is an awakening place.

It helps you find your creative life-force, your deeper truth, your secret purpose.

This world within your mind is a sacred landscape, a dimension of your thoughts and your feelings, to be explored like a great adventurer seeking hidden treasure in every cave, forest, and hideaway...

Bringing your focus back to your breath.

Let yourself continue exploring in ways you may not have before.

Let yourself delve more deeply into these ascended places.

Who do you meet along the way?

Have you met another spirit guide or ascended master who comes to teach you a lesson of healing and spiritual wisdom?

Do you have any specific places that you feel more draw to in this unique universe?

Wherever you are in your flight, give yourself a moment to see if you can find your castle again from this point of view.

Can you tell where you are on the map of your mind?

Are there secret tunnels and portals that will lead you right back to your castle?

Begin to find your way back to the castle now, breathing steadily and slowly along the way.

You can see it, and it feels far, but you have the ability to fly.

It won't take long to get there.

You are feeling more peaceful now and ready to fall fast asleep.

Your journey through the kingdom has shown you much and given you mush to appreciate.

You follow your original path back to the mirror where you first began.

Down, down, down the stone steps of the castle, like you are unwinding...

As you come to the mirror again, you see your eyes again, your face, your body.

You see your outfit.

It may have changed, and that's okay.

Or perhaps, after flying through your inner world, you are ready to take on a new form.

How do you want to dress now, as you prepare for a wholesome night of gentle, peaceful rest?

What would feel best to you right now after feeling the freedom of flight?

Take a few moments and breaths to see yourself in the castle mirror…

Now, you are ready.

You can now retire in your inner kingdom, in the castle of your dreams and imagination.

Not far from your looking glass is a large bed, fit for a queen or king.

It has the softest sheets and blankets, the deepest most relaxing pillows, and it is all for you, waiting for you, warm and inviting.

You walk over and climb your way up to the large mattress, tucking your legs under the covers, feeling silk against your skin.

You can finally rest after a long flight and journey around your kingdom.

As you snuggle in, long, heavy velvet curtains are pulled closed around the bed, wrapping you in comfort and deep, luxurious peacefulness.

You are free to disappear into your dreams now.

Your work is done.

You are here to rest all the way, deep into the world of the unconscious…

Release your breath...feel held by the magic of your castle, your kingdom, your inner world... you can fly anywhere you want, even all the way into your dreams.

You are floating into your dreams now, soft and serene, high up in your castle, safe, wrapped in velvet and silk...

Dream that you are flying over your kingdom again...peacefully, serenely, calmly...sweet dreams.

6. Cleanest Water

There once was a young knight named Pip, and Pip admired his queen. The Queen of Alanstar was one of the fairest women in the land. She had a mature demeanor, but creamy white skin, and long-flowing, silky black hair that seemed to envelop her throne. After the King passed many moons ago, the Queen ruled the land with a fair amount of care.

One day, the Queen summoned Pip to her throne room. The young knight bowed to his queen.

"What do you desire?" he asked.

"Good afternoon, my dear knight. I'm currently low on drinking water, and the knights who normally bring it to me are taking the day off."

Pip scratched his head a bit. There was plenty of water around. But before he could ask, the Queen answered for him.

"I drink the water from the peak of the Wellspring Mountain. At its tip, the cleanest, clearest water known to man resides. They say a fairy lives on top of the mountain, purifying the water. As it goes down the mountain, it becomes a little less pure, but still drinkable. However, I desire only the cleanest water the land has to offer. Could you give me a pail of it?"

Pip nodded. All his work for the Queen so far had been to mop up the castle, or to change her bed covers. This was something that maybe, just maybe, she'd reward him with.

The Queen handed him an empty pail, complete with a lid. This golden pail had some jewels in its rims, and it looked a little tacky, but shimmered, nonetheless. Pip immediately set forth after some preparations. He put everything on his trusted steed, Pap. Pap was a beautiful white horse who served him well in the few years he had been a night. With Pap by his side, Pip told him to giddy-up, and they were off, away from the castle's stables and to the unknown.

The Wellspring Mountain was not too far from the Kingdom of Alanstar. Its water, minerals, and wildlife all nourished the kingdom quite well. With that said, there was still a bit of travel before he made it to the kingdom, so Pip trotted down the field, seeing all the sights.

And so, their journey up the Wellspring Mountain began. The sound of the stream brought some relief, calming Pip's racing mind. Despite the climb, this task seemed safe. The scariest threat Pip faced so far was black bear that lapped up some water out of the mountain, but that bear just looked at Pip and paid no mind.

The water seemed to have a calming effect towards nature, and Pip and Pap stopped a few times to taste the mountain's water. It was already so clear, clean, and tasty. The Queen must have been really picky about her water.

Despite the initial climb being a bit of a breeze, the mountain soon began to steepen. There was a point where Pap made a sad whinney, unable to go any further. Pip hopped off.

"You just stay here," he said to Pap. "And I'll handle the rest."

He tied Pap next to a stream, leaving some oats behind. Pip unloaded any unneeded gear he had expect for his mountain climb, keeping only the pail, his equipment needed to climb, and the corn that Pop gave him. It was a long piece of corn, and quite filling. He munched on a bit as he began his climb up.

Pip's heart beat a bit as he climbed up, going higher and higher, his axe sinking into the mountainside. The cool, fall day soon became one that was a bit chillier the higher he went. The cool breeze danced around his temple and made his teeth chatter a bit, but he continued to climb.

As he climbed, with only his thoughts to entertain him, his mind began wandering. He was a kid again, training with his friends, their swords connecting in a rhythm that made him smile as he thought about it some more.

At the time, both him and his friend, Jaq, who since had departed for the Kingdom of Pio, always declared their love for the queen. "I'll be the queen's bodyguard!" Pip declared.

"No, I will," Jaq countered, and they continued to fight.

Pip chuckled as he climbed onward. He guessed this fight was still going on, even if Jaq had long since left the kingdom.

Pip continued his ascent, the temperature growing a bit colder and colder but he still persevered. He could see his skin reddening, and a bit of snot ran down his nose, but he still climbed. The queen would love him for this; he just knew it!

After what seemed like an eternity, he could see the top. Pip climbed straight to the top, and there, at the apex of the mountain, he saw something that made his eyes widen.

It was a beautiful hot spring. Steam rose from it, the heat immediately ridding himself of any potential frostbite he may have had. So, these were the legendary hot springs where the kingdom got his water. Here, the water was at its purest. It was hot, but free from any dirt, toxins, and packed filled with minerals needed to keep the body going.

Pip filled up his own canteen with some of the spring water, as he'd try it himself. Then, he began filling up the pail with the water. Soon, the pail was filled up, and he screwed the lid on. The water was safe and secure, and the way down was always better than the way up. Pip was about to make his way down, when he realized something.

This was probably going to be a once in a lifetime opportunity. Why couldn't he relax a bit? Pip took off his clothes and hopped into the hot springs. The water was that perfect balance of hot, but not too scalding. He felt the minerals kiss his skin, and the steam cleanse him of anything dirty he had on it. He let himself drift off a bit, almost falling asleep at the mercy of the springs. Ah.

"Hey!"

Pip opened his eyes. In front of him, a woman the size of a ruler floated above him, translucent wings flapping. She had crystal blue eyes, hair the color of a mountain snow, and a frown on her face.

"I spent all the time purifying the water, and yet, here is a man who dares to dirty himself in the springs. You should be ashamed of yourself."

Pip rubbed his eyes. Maybe he was just seeing things, but in front of him was a

"Fairy!" he exclaimed. He stood up and hopped out, and the fairy fluttered to where he was.

"Of course," the fairy said. "I am the Great Pixie, and I clean up all the water. But the water won't be too clean if you contaminate it. It's going to take me hours to purify it again! You should be ashamed of yourself. I ought to turn you into a mountain toad!"

Pip gasped. "I'm sorry," was all he could mutter. "I've traveled for so long, just to fetch a pail for my queen, and I wanted to take a break."

The Great Pixie nodded. "I don't blame you, but don't do it again. Gee, though. Fetching a pail for your queen? That sounds like a whole lot of work. Is she paying you well?"

Come to think of it, Pip shook his head. "She gives me payments for cleaning her room and for doing tasks, but it's just enough to eat and nothing more."

"Then why do you do it?" the pixie asked.

Pip scratched his chin. "I do it because I love my queen."

"Yeesh," the Pixie uttered, fluttering around Pip as she shook her head. "You do realize that she isn't going to 'return the favor,' if you get what I mean, just because you did something nice for her."

"Buzz off," Pip said. "I know what I'm doing."

The Pixie shook her head again. "Men, I swear. I'm glad I'm a pixie and not one of you humans. Anyway, I suppose you should be going. Go serve your queen or whatever."

Pip opened his eyes. He was back taking a dip in the hot springs. As he stood up, he looked for all signs of the pixie. However, she was gone.

"Did I fall asleep?" he muttered. It seemed so real. The fluttering of the wings, the sassy attitude, it all seemed to happen not too long ago in a plane that resembled reality. And yet, here he was, just a fool who almost drowned in the hot springs.

With that, he put his clothes back on, grabbed his pail and canteen, and began the journey down. As expected, it was a cakewalk. He sipped from the canteen when he was about halfway down. It tasted crystal clear and as he drank it, it felt like the water was washing everything unclean from his body until what was left was a crystal-clear interior.

Pip soon reached the bottom, and there, he met Pap again and began his journey back to the kingdom. The sun began to set as he made his way to the castle. Soon, he was back at the throne room.

"I see you are back," the Queen said. "I thought you may have fallen off." She chuckled a bit as he laid the pail at her feet. She opened the pail and sipped from it.

Pip smiled. "So, my lady, what do I get for doing all that work for you?"

The queen tapped her foot. "Well, our budget is a bit low, but I'll try to compensate you soon. Otherwise, your work here is done."

Pip sighed. "Is there anything else you could give me?"

An awkward air filled the room. Finally, the queen opened her mouth, and the words did not calm Pip.

"Not that I know of. Anyway, I'll be returned to my quarters. See you in the morrow."

With that, she retreated, and Pip was left in an empty throne room. He accomplished the task, and the queen seemed satisfied, and yet Pip had a hole as empty as that pail would soon be when the queen was thirsty.

The pixie's words echoed in his ear. Perhaps the queen wasn't meant for him. He was much younger, and had much less power, and the queen just saw him as her errand boy.

These thoughts danced around his head as he went to bed. He closed his eyes, and despite having a bit of trouble falling asleep, the fatigue of the day soon caught up to him. He fell into a dark, dreamless, descent into sleep.

When he woke up, his stomach growled, already hungry for breakfast. He reached into his satchel and saw that he had a bit of corn to him. He munched on it, and as he did so, a knight entered his quarters. "Pip, your Highness needs you," he said.

Pip finished the corn, and then looked at the cob. With a sigh, he got dressed, but rather than go to the queen's quarters, he instead walked to the stables. Pap looked at him, yawned, and accepted his ride with ease. Pip galloped out of the kingdom and into the countryside, where he swore a fairy was chasing him. But as he looked back, there was nothing. Fairies were not real, at least, he didn't think so.

Pip traveled for what seemed like forever, and then he eventually stopped at the cornfield that lied in front of him. There, he saw Pop, tending to the corn. She picked a few ears as Pip went closer to her.

He approached Pop, and she turned around and smiled. Pip smiled back, their awkward smiles mixing well together.

7. The Sweet Surrender

Get ready to fall asleep tonight with a guided sleep meditation and story that will help you relax in sweet surrender. At the end of summer has marveled humanity for centuries as these delicate yet Hardy creatures letter their way from the northeastern seaboard of the United States - as far as Mexico to seek respite from the cold winter. In this story, you will be able to travel along on this great migration before falling into a deep and healing sleep as you get cozy and dive into your sleep ritual. You may let go of your day and find your chest, heart, and lungs feeling lighter, imagining the lightness of being that a monarch butterfly enjoys throughout its life. As you sink into your bed and let your eyelids flutter closed before resting heavily upon your tired eyes inhaling and exhaling. As you tune into your breath, slowing it down, and as you inhale, you visualize the words; I am on the backs of your eyelids and exhale as the words light and carefree appear like a cursive neon-lit sign and inhaling. You see the words I am and then exhale to understand the terms letting go. This deep breath creates a rhythm, a soft and comfortable tempo that matches the gentle flutter of monarch butterflies' velvety wings. She glides above the golden sands of a barrier island at summers.

She is your guide on this journey, and you deeply trust her as young as she may be. She has been born with a roadmap and plans, just like you have been born with a roadmap and strong pull of intuition to guide you towards experiences. And people are meant to be a part of the tapestry of your life. This glorious monarch lands of harm the wet sand that now glitters like tiny golden topaz and diamond gemstones her feet. Taste the briny waters that I've washed the shore and naturally say and protected from the seagulls. Now feasting as her glorious black dots and stripes, orange and white pattern indicates to pray that she is poisonous to consume. So she is free to explore fearlessly and without a care and just as you may recall times in your life. When the Sun's warmth gave you energy and awakened you in a new day, the monarch butterfly no absorbs heat from the Sun that rises over the horizon. So she may begin her great migration southerly to escape the harshness of winter. You can experience all the sensations in this beautiful and safe mental state between your waking and sleeping life. This butterfly feels the comforting warmth from the Sun and the intuitive poll and understanding of where she must go, and you relish in her certainty. How she can commit to part of the journey without concern about the final destination, the migration is all about answering the call one day at a time for this monarch one flap of her papery wings.

At a time and just like you have transformed into different physical versions of yourself, the metamorphosis of this monarch from caterpillar to butterfly gives you a sense of relief, and growth and transformation are not just a conscious decision. They are often a requirement to serve me, and the greatest of growth may flow if you listen and tune in to your intuition and needs. Gently and calmly accepting this is part of being alive, and as the Sun begins to rise higher above the horizon and glittering sapphire sea illuminating the sky. The temperature starts to increase the air becomes misty from a haze of silvery-blue morning fog that coats. The warm golden sands the ocean is at its warmest temperature after months of intense July and August heat. Long days of sunlight have transformed it into a heated saltwater bath. The monarch takes one last solo pass across the shoreline. The same shore she may return to come springtime, she is full of energy and life vivacity. As brilliant as the vibrancy of her velvety orange hue wings. She flutters inland towards a pine home that has been faded by the salty air. Lands upon potted zinnias in shades of fuchsia and purple and marigold yellow. She was sitting in the nectar that coats our black feet with its intoxicating fragrance filling up.

Other monarchs join her, also getting in their nourishment before the great flight southward begins. Then just like the streams of an orchestra that is warming up for a performance, the first of the swarm of butterflies begin to take to the cerulean blue skies going higher and higher. You can feel the splendor of what this is like this easy ascent towards. The sky fluttering up and up as a wind assists their plight like a summers wind hitting the sails of a boat out at sea-salty air has the slightest net. The cut through the otherwise warm morning's temperature is a gentle battle between the heat of the Sun and autumns chill. But for now, the warmth winds out during daylight hours, and the monarch butterflies inherently understand this and use this particular time to begin their epic journey. You feel how freeing it has the support of the breeze beneath your monarch guides wings that seamlessly Blyde forward, able to travel up to 100 miles or 160 kilometers. A day relies on the gold and sun to activate and support their journey; the monarchs travel above the visto of lush emerald green marshes. Waterways along the Seaboard and human-made homes that scatter the landscape below the trees are beginning to change colors.

While predominantly a verdant green, it is as if the forest below is speckled with hops of gold, magenta, and orange leg, a mystical speckled egg from a distance. It is so natural and comfortable to appreciate the splendor of the planet below, and you take it in the brightness of the experience. The wonder of being such a small yet resilient life-form a flock of seagulls flies in the opposite direction sharing the open skies that are so vast. Yet offer a sense of community for all air-bound creatures. They have been gifted with skills that take them away from the land-bound and water-bound species below and right. Now relish their ability to soar the landscape below becomes meditative a continual kaleidoscope of life basking in the afternoon's Sun. You think back to all the times in your life as a child or even in the dreamscapes of your sleeping life where you imagined what it would feel like to fly how wondrous. It would be to escape the strong pull of gravity and to look at the planet from a new vantage point as you inhale and exhale looking through the eyes and living the experience of this monarch butterfly. You intake all the sensations of this journey what it is like to be. So light and feathery and yet so durable and determined with a set direction and end goal to be so beautiful and vibrant with velvety soft wings. That seems so fragile and again can endure four months of light during migration to appear.

So captivating and delicate and yet simultaneously convey a sense of danger to all potential predators how perfect it is to be a butterfly. You relish in this protection, and as you go deeper and deeper within, you realize that you, too, are part of perfection. You are here to learn to grow and to transform, and you are doing that every single new day you're opening yourself to new experiences.

You're tending to your basic needs for relaxation and respite at the end of the day. You may take this moment to celebrate you to celebrate the spectacular moment in time that you had this shift. You answered this call to work towards being your best self to aligning yourself with the greater good for you to listening to that intuitive voice that begins. As a whisper and can become as loud as necessary until you hear your inner voice. On this light, this intuitive journey of the monarch butterflies you vow to go deeper and deeper within does their ender and listen to your truth. To the guidance that the universe is always offering to you like two dials in your heart center reminiscent of an old radio dial, you may tune in to the right frequency and with the other dial. You may tune up the volume until you hear what needs to be heard, and you're doing so very well feeling so relaxed.

The day is beginning to fade into the night, and the kaleidoscope of monarch butterflies are slowing down and light during the hottest point of the day the Monarchs were able to ascend. As high as 10,000 feet or 3,000 meters above the Earth's surface as the temperature drops. The Sun lowers beyond the horizon the last of the liquid orange waves of light spanning the landscape in deciduous and evergreen trees. Below the Monarchs begin to lower intuitively aware they may drop out of the sky if the temperature decreases to significantly gently gliding down beneath the shadows of the trees flattering as autumn leaves on a night wind. The air clean and Kris the aromas of the forest floor and behind trees swirling up through the spaces between feathery branches becoming more fragrant. The further and further down towards the ground, the Monarchs have loved your monarch guide leads. The swarm of butterflies settling among the damp branches of a pine tree all settling Emirati branches their feet is taking in the sticky pine pitch's aroma. You feel what it's like to nestle among the owls and squirrels and deer and birds and rabbits that I've all gotten cozy for the night. I ready to surrender to their tiredness. It is the completion of another day and for the monarch butterflies. This journey will continue for months, with each day finding them.

A first-time glimpse has new parts of the continent, and each night will bring a comfortable retreat or respite. You may think of your life in the same way no day is ever the same, even if you are doing the same things. You are different each day the circumstances change. So many new things await being discovered by you. Each night welcomes you like a gentle hug and unique sanctuary offering you sleep—an escape from your toils and challenges of each day. In the months that come like centuries ago, people will await the arrival of the swarms of butterflies seeking escape from the cold their iconic wings, bringing them to a new place. How spreading beauty across the land monarch butterflies serving as nature's most beautiful hand-painted canvas. Just as they are awaited, there are people in the future that welcome and await you as you grow and transform on your journey. You are free to explore the intuitive urges and a divine inner voice within us all and with a peaceful hum of the forest. The sacred sound of crickets and a babbling brook you are welcome to find piece and rasp it to find sleep to get cozy and relaxed to get all the rest. It would be best if you continued to grow and transform - let the blank canvas of your dreams awaits you tonight to be painted with the same beauty that accompanies the journey. You have earned this moment you deserve this. You're worthy of the peace and stillness that accompanies you as you are ready to let go and slip into a dream world of bliss. I am going to count you down to this place for healing sleep feeling so heavy and relaxed ten nine eight seven six by three to one finding rest finding stillness. Finding sleep, it's time to dream away goodnight.

8. The Childhood Blanket

While asleep easily and quickly with our guidance. Sleep meditation, you may find comfort and safety as these feelings wrap around you like a childhood blanket and allow you to trust in yourself. In your life, at times in life, there may win out over love and joy like a switch that turns on a light. So - may you turn on an internal switch to illuminate the dark corners. Where anxiety and fear and self-doubt. May lurk it may not be easy, but it is most certainly possible I would like to welcome you to Michelle Sanctuary. You are listening to healing sleep meditation. Your okay, and it's all good. This talk down will help you make peace with your path with all the challenges of the past.

All that may be currently troubling you right now will allow you to relax and unwind deeply. Let it all go right now; let it all just go you don't need it. You never did. You don't need to hold on to anything. You may even visualize the gates of a levee opening and releasing a reservoir of water into the sea, allowing all your thoughts and concerns to flow out and merge with something vast and expansive. Suddenly your problems seem quite small it is no longer your responsibility to keep all of this is because you are okay. It is all good, yes, you are okay, and it is all good and perhaps. You may remember a time in your life when you are scared are not feeling well. We're comforted by someone who loves you very much in the safety of an embrace are imagining the fingers of a loved one.

One gently brushing your hair away from your face; you may hear this kind whisper. How true-time proved it to be right it's going to be okay you are going to be okay. Nothing stays. The same forever, this too shall pass you are okay. You are going to be just fine. Maybe you don't have it all figured out. Perhaps you don't know much about it. This adulting business and you're tired of trying to figure it all out. But you need not worry or figure it out tonight. You know you don't even need to completely figure it out in this lifetime at all because no one has completely figured out life. As it unfolds is a continuous series of lessons an education that you may learn from, and if you don't learn the first time, you will surely be given time. Time again, one experience after the next to be given another chance to try and learn the lesson time to figure it out. There is plenty of time ahead; there is not a deadline for you that pressure may just put more anxiety into a toolbox that should be full of tools. An arsenal of all your strengths and wisdom intuition and creativity should be allowed every inch of space; those worries are not worth space.

They try to take up, and you deserve to have love and self-acceptance and nurture yourself and to feel nurtured by those around you. Because you are doing just fine, you are okay. It is all good, and your mind and emotions indicate how you feel and what stories you may tell yourself about yourself. You may change the story; you may readjust the way you process and think about things. You may make a choice right now to feel good to feel safe to say to yourself I am okay. And I am doing the best that I can do, given all the experiences. I have been given I am trying I can fall and get back up again. I can listen to my inner voice and guidance. I can acknowledge that deep down, I have my inner compass to guide me. I can trust that I can find stillness deep within I can seek a sanctuary to heal my wounds. To get healthy again so I can go into the world and thrive, I am doing the best I can for myself and for forgiving others. Because forgiveness is the best gift, I may give to myself and to those who have hurt or disappointed me or just let me down. Because it is all part of the human experience, you are only human. So is everyone else around you, and it's okay, and it's all good, our life is all about choices. We are the ones in charge of these choices. So right now, in your sanctuary and within the safety of your mind. You may go deeper and deeper within and go to the steady warm flow of peace that comes.

You may even let these words drift across the movie screens on the backs of your dark closed eyelids as you sudden. These mantras and messages way up here in any style font let any way on the screen that you desire I choose to forgive. I want to let go. I want to recognize what is in my control and to surrender what is not I want to believe that. I came to this life to learn and that the hardships I experienced are meant to bring me closer to what I need and desire. I choose to trust I want to honor me. As used to let go of pride and my ego for the sake of love and happiness. I want to listen to my intuition. I want to listen to everything and everyone around me. So I may learn and grow I want empathy I'd want to recognize my strengths and embrace it. I want to be me. I choose to let myself shine; I choose to love myself. I choose to be brave; it's used to acknowledge that everyone around me has been afraid of dealing with their limitations. Their fears, I choose to recognize my fear. So I may overcome it, I choose to deal with myself I choose to honor my past but embrace the present. I choose to connect with others. I choose to connect with my presence so that I may be led to the future. I most desire I decide to accept that I have a finite time that is precious in this life to do all the things. I need to do and to say all the things I need to say I choose to try; I choose to believe I choose to be okay with everything right now.

I choose to feel okay because I am okay, and it is all good. As you feel your body relaxing, your muscles are melting. All that you have been carrying with you all that as a wage you down may be released from your body. You no longer need to take all that weight. Maybe right now, you are just becoming aware of all that has been haunting you and holding you back. You may let go of these blocks to your creativity into your journey because you are okay. It is all good. You may not know your direction; you may not know what you want, but it is okay. If this is so, then your current life's purpose is to discover what you want, and if or when you find out this, you are ready and able to go. After what you wish to because it is yours and you can do this, you've got this. You are doing just fine. Even when you feel like you are not enough, you may trust me. As I say this, you are enough; you are everything you need to be every step has gotten to where you are right now. So you need not live and regret it because you are here directly. Right here on the right path, and you know this because you took the time to find a sanctuary and to connect, you took the time to come here.

Just accept that everything is okay. Everything is just as it should be right now, and you are doing all you need to be doing just breathing in and out. Because one conscious breath is a meditation, you're able to take another conscious breath inhaling and believing. In the mystical powers, the cause synchronicity that caused things to come together at the right time. In the right place that brings you to a state of wonder and faith. Right now, the trust begins with you was believing in yourself; it just takes the tiniest spark of belief right now to ignite a fire that will burn within you. Because it is all right thinking about how many problems you have already solved in this life, in this year, in this month in the week and even today, how many things you had overcome even when you did not want to be faced with them. Every time you overcame, you instill this deep memory that you can do this that you have already done hard things. Save prevailed. You're still here in any fears you may have about the end of life. May drift away because all you need to do is live each day to the fullest to make the most out of every moment. Every connection with those that you love that you may allow in new influences. People that foster your growth and believe in you realize this right now say to yourself I am okay, I will be okay.

It is all good, and I am right, and this is good, and everything will be okay, and being alright does not mean perfect it. It does not mean things are how you want them to be all the time. It does not mean that everything is figured out that you have mastered the art of being an adult. But you've figured out everything about life, maybe you know even less now. Then you thought you knew before, and that is okay because being okay is a choice of acceptance and surrender. Being okay means, you are choosing your happiness and ease of being and balanced mind over unmet expectations and disappointment. We are all disappointed at times, and that is okay disappointment serve as an opportunity to tune you into what you want to light a fire in your heart to motivate. You to empower you to be brave enough to say perhaps at first in the chambers of your mind. Later to the world beyond you, I want this; I need this; I can no longer be afraid. I choose to do what it takes to get what I need and desire. May be right, we lose things a little bit at a time because it is all good. You may realize how much better it feels to just surrender like a sea turtle riding the waves of a gentle turquoise sea you too may ride along. Let go doing fine, recognizing what is in your control and what is not. You can control your feelings. You can manage your thoughts; you can control what choices you make; you can control how you express what you need and desire. You're very good at doing this.

You may be brave. You may accept that your feelings matter your thoughts matter. It's okay to have opinions that sometimes are intense. But sometimes, don't feel right. You are learning to embrace and acknowledge what they are. You are choosing to shine a light on what can be healed. Rather than burying it deep within and those voices that you sometimes hear, perhaps those who have influenced you caused you to have doubts within yourself. They may be silenced; maybe it is your voice creating chatter a causes anxiety and self-doubt that may now be released these voices. Never felt good anyway, so I hold on to them just as you would turn a radio dial when a song comes on that you do not enjoy. So - may you now change the thoughts in your mind surrender and drift towards. And all the things that make you feel good about yourself to think about everything that you love most about being you about something. You have done for others that make you feel good about the love you have been able to think about the bonds. You have formed in your life, reflecting on the chances. You have been given the times you have listened to your intuition and indeed allowed stillness to grant you the insight to guide your life, trusting that this voice is always.

There the useful inner guide that is you that has always been you the part of you that has existed throughout your entire life. You may find that voice growing louder, and like a watercolor painting left out in gentle spring rain, these thoughts become like watercolors that melt into your dreaming life. So you may continue to dream tonight and have guidance that will allow you to wake up feeling motivated and inspired. Because it's okay, you are okay and will be alright tomorrow and the days that come ahead. It is all good and feeling this lightness of being like a kite sailing across a clear sky. You are now free to cross the unique bridge into your dreaming life. This is a sacred time that comes at least once a day wheN you drift and surrender to the deep sleep and healing and empowering dreams that await you. You may go across this bridge, letting yourself float through the misty air. In the most ethereal of transitions going deeper and deeper down towards sleep towards dreams that show the acceptance. You have of being okay a feeling good about where you are with who you are because you are okay. It is all good, and I am going to count you down towards a restorative night of sleep that you have earned. So rightfully deserve where you may take in the lessons of the day. Explore the possibilities for two more lettings go of my voice letting go of your waking life 10 9 8 7 6 5 4 3 2 1 finding bliss finding healing finding peace finding out that it's all right it's time to dream away the excellent night.

9. Floating Across a Pale Blue Sky

Sometimes, all you need is to feel far from all of your cares and worries.

Sometimes, all you need is to glide through life on a serene cloud, floating across a pale blue sky.

If you have ever been on an airplane ride and looked out the window, then you have probably noticed the ethereal world above the clouds.

It is so calm and relaxing, high off the ground, and far away from all of the stress of life.

Have you ever taken a ride in a hot air balloon?

Have you ever been lifted off the ground slowly, like you were being carried by a gentle giant to a restful place?

Your journey into peacefulness and relaxation will begin on the ground, preparing for your journey of slow and tender flight, as you crawl slowly through the clouds in a comfortable basket.

Begin your ascent first by lying down in a comfortable position.

If your body needs to be adjusted at all to help you for the most comfort in this space, make those adjustments now before you enter a place of total stillness.

You are going to be carried away on the air, firstly through your breath.

Your breath will align you with your inner harmony and balance.

Your breath will help fill you with the peacefulness you desire and help you release all of the cares and worries you may be carrying around with you right now.

Every inhale is a beautiful source [of comfort, refreshment, and light.

Every exhale is a letting go, a release of tension, a movement closer to restful relaxation.

Breathe here for a few moments.

Connect to your body.

Connect to your feelings.

Connect to the sense of relief from your breath...

You are here to feel free from the world of deadlines and agendas.

You are here to only exist within yourself and your deeper sense of true peace and balance.

This practice of connecting to your physical body through your breath, and your spiritual essence through your creative mind, is what will help you to refresh your life-force energy and feel fully healed, refreshed and connected to your inner soul.

Your only purpose now is just to float through a heavenly landscape.

Underneath your body, you begin to feel the softness of grass on a majestic hillside.

It is a bright and beautiful, sunny day.

As you look up into the sky, you can see that it is full of the most glorious, puffy, white clouds.

You look over now and see the basket just walking distance away—the basket that will carry you far off into the heavens.

You are eager to go over to it and witness the gigantic balloon rise up off the ground, full of the hot air that will lift you up.

The basket is easy for you to climb into a much larger than you would have thought.

There is enough room inside for you to lie down in any direction.

The balloon is airing up while you are climbing inside.

It is starting to lift off of the grassy earth and align with the basket, to float over and hover above it.

You can feel yourself feeling elated but calm—excited, but relaxed.

Your path is up and up and up, and there is no other landscape, but the clouds on high.

You will get there soon.

Your balloon is almost ready to lift you up and all you have to do when the time comes is pull on the cord to send you off the ground.

Inhale deeply, slowly pulling fresh air into your lungs...and exhale gently out.

Again, inhale slowly and steadily, gathering all of the hot air you will need to soar high up in the clouds...and exhale.

Breathe out all of the cares and worries that will weigh you down.

Breathe away all of the tension that will keep your balloon on the ground...

You are ready, and your balloon is ready.

It's time to pull the cord and feel your ascent.

The cord is easy to pull.

It feels effortless as you give it a tug and release hot air into the giant balloon above your head.

The river is full of life, and it flows smoothly, cutting across the land as far as the eye can see, the sunlight of the day glistening on its surface.

The river becomes smaller and smaller as you float higher and higher, taking a deep breath in and exhaling gently...

You look to the west, and you see a great, wide forest that pushes far across the land.

The higher you go, the smaller the trees become, the wood of the branches and trunks disappearing behind the green foliage.

The tops of the trees, which once seemed so close, are now at a great distance from your hot air balloon.

You can feel the journey getting steadily closer to the clouds...

You look out of the basket to the south, and you see fields and meadows reaching far across the land, sewing a patchwork quilt of land as far as your eye can see to the south.

The lands of the farmers, the cattle, the goats and the sheep—the land of food that grows, of harvests and abundance from the fertile soil.

This land will stretch out for miles more, as your balloon gets ever higher, and can see that much farther across the land.

You look out to the north and are much higher now.

You begin to see the curve of the Earth from this height and feel completely restful as you look to the North Star, already visible from this height in the sky.

You have ascended to the atmosphere of the cloud world, and it is here that you will find your greatest peacefulness and comfort.

It is here that you can let all of your worries and cares drift off and away from you, falling back to the earth as you drift through the clouds...

Look around you as you inhale deeply and exhale smoothly.

You are completely surrounded by puffs of white moisture.

They look like giant cotton balls piled together in beautiful mounds of softness.

Your basket is moving slowly, but you feel the momentum of your balloon as it wafts on the breeze of the high atmosphere.

You have no trouble breathing here.

You can take deep, fulfilling breaths.

You can feel totally relaxed as you inhale and exhale from this point in the sky...

Breathe now as you let in the magnificent scenery of an all-white horizon fill your soul.

Breathe into this place of total calm and serenity.

Let the clouds high above the earth; comfort you.

You are warm here.

You are safe.

You have enough oxygen to breathe.

All you have to do is take in the majesty of this place.

The whole world above the clouds looks like a tundra of snow and ice for thousands of miles.

It looks angelic and full of bright light, the light from the sun reflecting off of the cloud faces.

Beneath the clouds is the whole landscape of the world you know—the world where you eat, sleep, work, love...

Let it come fully into your thoughts.

As you let it take shape in your thoughts, turn it into something you can hold in your hand, a physical object that represents this worry or stress...

It could be a heavy bag of sand that represents the weight that you feel from your work or your home life.

It could be a dollhouse to symbolize how you feel about your home or your living space.

It could be a person that has been upsetting you or weighing you down. Anything is possible from this place within your mind.

Do not judge yourself for how it comes up or how it forms.

Simply allow it to take shape so that you can hold it in your hands…

Notice the clouds again and the atmosphere you are floating again.

Reminding yourself of your stress may have brought up those feelings for you again.

Look out to the clouds.

You are here in a hot air balloon, free to just release the pain you are suffering, free to align with your highest consciousness and internal vibration of light…

Here you are, high above the clouds, facing your current anxiety or worry.

You are holding it in your hands, and you are ready to let it go.

You can hold it over the side of the balloon and prepare to let it go.

You are not hurting it, whatever it is.

It is a symbolic release of what has been holding you back from your relaxation and relief.

It is a symbolic action to cut the cords with your tension, worry, and doubt…

Hold the symbolic object over the edge and promise to let go of everything right here, right now.

You have no reason to hold onto this part of your life anymore.

You have no reason to doubt yourself.

You have no reason to fear to let go of this issue or these fears.

It is time.

Here, high above the clouds, it is time for you to say farewell to this part of your life.

It serves no purpose.

It only causes distress and discomfort.

Let it go.

Let it fall far away, through the clouds to wherever it must go.

Resolve to know that you are free of it.

Release it fully and take a nice, long breath in through your nose.

Hold your breath here for a moment, like you were holding the object over the side of the basket...and release the breath, letting it flow away from you.

Notice the serene landscape around you, unfolding as far as your eye can see...

You are safe here.

You are free.

You have released your discomfort.

You can now relax a little more and let yourself delve more deeply into your unconscious thoughts and dreams.

Here in the heavens, high above the soft, cotton-like clouds, you can prepare for your ascent farther and deeper into dreamland.

You will not return to the Earth tonight.

Tonight, you will continue to float high above the ground in your hot air balloon and find all of the relief you have been looking for.

Exercise

Monkey Moment

TIME TO READ: 2 MINUTES

TIME TO DO: 8 MINUTES

This exercise is a great technique for managing anxiety. Try imagining the anxiety inside you as a cute little monkey that worries about being left behind. Perhaps you could engage the monkey and have some compassion for its fears. Understand that you are much wiser than the monkey, so you can listen to its concerns and also choose how you feel about them.

1. Go to a favorite trail, a peaceful area, or simply take a walk in your neighborhood before you go to school. Set your timer for 8 minutes. Begin by walking slowly, placing one foot in front of the other—heel to toe.

2. While walking, repeat the positive self-mantra "May my monkey have peace."

3. As you say this, imagine the monkey calming down and resting on your back.

10. A Forty-something-year-old Woman

Darlene was a forty-something-year-old woman who had spent her entire life doing everything that she knew she was supposed to do.

She woke up every morning at six to feed her dogs and her cat, she made breakfast for her children and her husband, and she fixed a pot of morning coffee. When everyone was fed, she would clean their plates away, tidy up the kitchen, and help everyone get ready for their day. Then, it was off to school.

Darlene would then head into the office to work until the school day was over. She would then go pick up her children, bring them home, feed them a snack, and escort them to their after-school activities like soccer, dance, and swim lessons.

When everyone got home in the evening, Darlene would fix up a supper, feed everyone, and then clean all of the dishes when everyone was done eating. She would then clean up everyone's book bags and shoes, tidy up any other messes that had been made that day, and then sit down to watch thirty minutes of television before bed.

On weekends, Darlene would do all of the same things except instead of going to school or work she would take her kids shopping, to sleepovers, or to their sports events. There was always something going on, and Darlene was always in charge of having to make sure that everything got done in time.

When she was in her early forties, Darlene realized that she was entirely miserable. After spending nearly two decades cleaning up after her family, preparing meals for them, and driving them around everywhere, Darlene realized that she was done.

She no longer cared to have the experience of doing everything herself, as it was beginning to take a toll on her. She found that every morning she would wake up depressed and dreading the day before her, and every night she would go to sleep sad and wishing that she could wake up to a brand-new life. This brought Darlene great guilt as she loved her family and loved caring for them, though she could no longer do it all by herself.

One day, Darlene was called into her boss's office in the middle of the afternoon. As she got up from her desk and headed toward her bosses office, Darlene tried to recall anything she may have done wrong that could result in her being talked to or written up by her boss.

Of course, she could not think of anything she had done wrong as Darlene was always very particular about doing everything properly and by the book. After all, she was great at doing what she knew was expected of her. When she reached her bosses office, Darlene's boss asked her to sit and offered to get her a beverage.

Darlene agreed and began sipping on the tea that her boss had brought her as she tried to understand what it was that she had been called in for. To her surprised, Darlene's boss offered her a promotion that came with a substantial raise and increased benefits compared to what she was already receiving.

Darlene was excited by the offer, but at the same time, she was miserable to realize that taking it meant that she would be committing to staying in this lackluster life that she was no longer getting joy from.

Before she knew what, she was doing, Darlene refused the promotion and instead put in her notice and quit her job. She went and cleared out her desk and left, never to look back again.

Darlene's family was surprised to learn that she had quit her job and had no intentions of going back. They were also surprised when she said that she would no longer make breakfast unless she felt like it, that everyone would need to find their own ways to their hangouts, and that the only thing Darlene would help with anymore was getting to sports events or homework.

At this point, her kids were old enough that they could walk, bike, or even drive themselves to their own events so she would no longer have to do it. In other words, Darlene was ready to start letting her children grow up and become young adults.

Asserting these boundaries meant that Darlene had great freedom in her life to do whatever it was that she pleased. She could sleep in, eat whenever she wanted, and even watch afternoon television shows that she had heard her friends talking about at the PTA meetings at her children's school for years.

Finally, Darlene got what it meant to slow down and just be, rather than to always have to be in motion doing everything in her power to please everyone else.

At first, Darlene's laid-back lifestyle was enjoyable as it offered her a great change of pace from what she was used to. Over time, however, it grew boring as she realized that she would always be doing nothing unless she did something to change that. As she did not want to spend her entire life bored, Darlene began looking into different hobbies and discovering new things that she liked.

One hobby she found that she was drawn to was making jewelry. Darlene found that not only did she enjoy making jewelry, but also that she was incredibly good at it, and that people often wanted to purchase her jewelry.

Darlene started out making jewelry as a hobby in the afternoons while she watched daytime television. She would make four or five new pieces per week, and inevitably every single piece would sell to someone that she knew.

Eventually, she started selling her jewelry online as this gave her the opportunity to sell even more.

Before she knew it, Darlene was making copious amounts of jewelry and selling them to friends, family, strangers online, and even stocking it in boutique stores around her town. She grew so excited to make jewelry that Darlene would excitedly get up in the middle of the night and sketch out new plans, or launch from bed in the morning ready to start crafting new creations.

Although it was a far cry from what she was used to, Darlene loved her new life of making and selling handmade jewelry.

Her children and husband liked it as well, as they began to realize that Darlene was happier and enjoying life once again. It took them some time to get used to Darlene not being available to help as often anymore, but in the end, they were all happy that Darlene had found her passion and that she was finally enjoying life after helping her family do the very same thing for so many years.

11. Hold the Key to Your Relief

You are alone in your bed or your space of comfort.

You are here to rest and relax.

There is nothing left to do now but just sink into the covers, melt into the mattress, and find relief in your body after a long day.

You are here to fully inspire total serenity, peace of mind, and relaxation.

Anything you need to do to find your most comfortable resting position do so now…

Take a moment to honor your body.

Find your stillness and your center.

Let go of any judgments you have about your body or the way it feels.

Simply notice the areas that are holding onto something or that have tension, and let it all flow out when you exhale.

Your body can begin to rest.

Underneath all of the layers of your day, your work, your relationships, your tasks or deadlines, there is just quiet space.

In this bedtime story, you are going to find a secret map that will take you to this place of quiet and release so that you can find a deeper comfort from within you.

You hold the key to your relief, and this guided meditation and bedtime visualization will take you there, one step at a time.

Your breath should start to become long...and slow...and steady.

Let it flow naturally.

Don't overthink your breathing.

Just allow it to transport you more deeply into your relaxed state of mind and body.

Your physical self has been at work all day.

Even if you weren't moving around all that much, if you had to sit down at your desk, or work from a seated position somewhere, your whole body has still worked hard.

Your mind has been hard at work, even when you are at play.

You are always thinking, weighing and calculating, observing, listening, processing.

You have all of the energy of thought radiating from your brain and from your body.

Now, you can begin to let your energy flow in longer, thicker waves.

You no longer need to be in a state of attention.

You are now free to sink into a state of total relaxation.

Help your body feel softer and more elastic with each inhale of breath, and each exhale of tension or any kind of thoughts or ideas that keep circling around.

Breathe it all out and come to a place of peace of mind...and body.

You are now in a more relaxed state of energy, and you can fall even deeper into your unconsciousness.

You are ready to take a journey farther than you have ever traveled before.

You are ready to discover your highest state of relief, your most sacred level of self-healing, finding your balance with every breath as you transcend space, time, and the material world.

Begin to see in your mind a bright light at the end of a long tunnel.

The tunnel is a part of your mind that takes you into a deeper layer of your consciousness.

You can float through the tunnel, like a seed on the wind, going closer to the light at the end, feeling yourself soften, and welcome the spiral of light that opens before you...

The tunnel is widening as you come fully into the light.

Feel it surround you, almost blinding you from what lies on the other side.

The light is so bright that it fills your whole being, penetrating your skin, and filling you with healing warmth and love.

You can feel it with every breath you inhale, the light filling your lungs, and circulating through your body.

As you exhale now, you will feel the brightness of the light normalize, opening your sight to see a great open meadow covered in soft green grass and flowers dancing on a soft breeze.

The air around you is crisp and clear, clean, and cool, but your body remains warm, safe, protected.

You can see a wide range of snow-capped mountains surrounding the meadow.

It is bright and open, full of possibilities.

You are here in this space, a place of your deeper mind.

You are free to explore this land, this mountain range, this secret world.

You feel an urge to explore in several directions, and you aren't quite sure where to begin.

There are many potential paths to explore, many ways you can go to find your deepest calm and relaxation.

If only you had a map, a map that could point you in the right direction, a map that would hold you close and give you everything you need to explore this place and guide you to your serenity.

As you ponder this, you feel a tingle in your palms.

Lifting up your hands, you notice that there are markings where there were none before.

The markings are starting to make sense.

A map is imprinted on your palms.

It shows you exactly where you need to go.

Your healing path is always in your hands, and all you have to do is trust yourself that you already know where you need to go to find inner harmony and peace.

The map on your hands is showing you a path to walk.

You look up at the mountains and the meadow, and you find the direction your hands are pointing you toward.

Follow the arrows of your inner mind.

Follow the way you are showing yourself to travel.

Walk in that direction, noticing the place you are and how it feels to have awareness in your deeper mind.

Inhale deeply and let out a long, slow breath.

Let your body remain relaxed, peaceful, serene, as your mind travels to these inner pathways.

Perhaps a fog thickens on your path, or maybe there is a soothing river flowing across your path.

Let the natural world of your mind unfold.

If you are uncertain of where to travel, look down at the map on your hands for guidance.

Trust your intuition to show you the path...

As you continue to breathe and follow your secret map forward, let yourself begin to seek even further down into your subconscious mind.

The landscape, the dreamscape, the world of your mind can become anything you want it to be.

Where is it leading you?

What is happening on your path as you follow the secret map of your soul and your mind?

Is it still comforting and pleasant?

Do you feel like your map has taken you on a darker road, a more shadowy path?

Are you still following the map of yourself to find where to go?

If you begin to feel like you are getting off the path, or if you feel like you are leading yourself into dark territory, that's okay.

Sometimes that can be exactly where you need to travel to heal your deeper self and your deeper mind.

If you need to get back on a lighter path, you can take a few soothing breaths in and out, and let the sun come out and beam bright, warm, healing light onto the shadows of your mind.

Let the map continue to show you the way you need to go.

Underneath the power of your journey lies the answer to where your inner harmony lives and breathes.

Somewhere the map of your consciousness is the answer to how to heal yourself on the deepest level.

Your secret map is always working with you to help you find your path.

Now, look down at the map on your hands.

Look to see if there is an 'X' that marks the end of your quest in this sacred wilderness deep within your mind.

Do you see it?

How are you going to get there?

How will the path take you to the 'X' on the map?

Looking around, can you see where you want to go?

Can you sense where that X is inside of this place?

Go there. Seek it out.

Find the X from the palm of your hand in the land of your mind, in the place of your soul and your subconscious.

Perhaps it is a very direct path.

Perhaps it is winding and bending.

Maybe you need to climb over a few obstacles here and there, or perhaps you encounter a challenge along the road.

Keep going.

When in doubt, look at the map on your hand.

Let it lead you to the X that marks the spot... (take several moments to search for it).

You are now around the spot where your final destination is laid.

You have found the ground where the 'X' is painted or etched on the earth or on a tree.

Perhaps it is carved in the rocks of the mountainside, or it could be less obvious and more like a feeling that you just know that this is the place.

What does this place look like?

How does it feel to be here?

How long did it take you to find it?

Inhale deeply, taking a long soothing breath of air into your body.

Hold it for a moment, and now exhale slowly, steadily letting the air leave you.

And inhale again, filling yourself with the feeling of discovery, the feeling of finding the spot on your map.

Exhale slowly, going deeper into your mind, deeper into your fullness and relaxed state.

Here is where your healing can begin, when you let go of all of the other spaces outside of you, when you seek out your 'X' on your inner map, as it guides you into the deepest points of growth and transformation, the deepest points of total relaxation and relief.

Here is where you can release judgment and critique.

Here is where you can enlist your power to resolve the hardest moments and the biggest challenges.

Let your body sink into this space.

Let your heart open to finding resolve so that you can feel at peace.

Your mind is made of thoughts and beliefs, attitudes, and emotions.

Your mind is also made of spirit, your spirit—the life force energy that gives you the secret map of your inner journey.

Your spirit aligns you with your purpose and the right path for you, directing you along the way, a new direction every day.

All you have to do is find your focus and follow the map to where your 'X' marks the spot.

This map has led you to a place of total peace and inner harmony.

You are here to rest, sleep, dream.

You are here to fall deeply into serenity and balance.

In the space, deep within your subconscious mind, you now see a door.

This door is familiar to you, and you know that it will lead you back home, back to the security of your warm bed, back to your whole body and mind.

When you walk through this door, all you have to do is rest.

All you have to do is sleep.

All you have to do is dream of where your secret map will lead you next.

Walkthrough the door...sink deeply into your mattress or cushions...go deeply into the dreamworld...until the next map leads you to where you need to be...

12. The Amazing Princess

Once upon a time there was a poor man who had had as many children as holes in a sieve and all the people in his village as godparents. When he was again born a son, he sat down on the road to ask the first best to be godfather. Then an old man in a gray cloak came to meet him, he asked, and he agreed and went to the baptism. As a baptismal gift, the old man gave the father a cow with a calf. That was born the same day as the boy and had a golden star on his forehead.

The boy grew older and bigger and the calf also grew, became a big bull and the boy led him every day to the mountain meadow. But the bull was able to speak, and when they were on the top of the mountain, the bull spoke: "Stay here and sleep, I want to find my own willow!" As soon as the boy fell asleep, the bull ran like lightning on the big one Sky meadow and eats golden star flowers. When the sun went down, he hurried back, woke the boy, and then they went home. So it happened every day until the boy was twenty years old.

One day the bull spoke to him: "Now sit between my horns, I carry you to the king. Demand from him a seven-meter-long iron sword and tell him that you want to save his daughter."

Soon they arrived at the castle. The boy dismounted, went to the king and said why he had come. He gladly gave the shepherd boy the required sword. But he had no hope of ever seeing his daughter again. Already many brave youths had tried in vain to rescue them, because a twelve-headed dragon had kidnapped them, and this lived far away, where nobody could get to. First, there was a high, insurmountable mountain on the way there, secondly, a wide and stormy sea, and third, the dragon lived in a castle of flame. If any one had succeeded in crossing the mountains and the sea, he would not have been able to penetrate through the mighty flames, and if he had succeeded, the dragon would have killed him.

When the boy had the sword, he sat down between the horns of the bull, and in no time they were before the great mountain. "Now we have to turn back," he said to the bull, for it seemed impossible for him to get across. But the bull said: "Wait a minute!", Put the boy on the ground, and as soon as that happened, he took a start and pushed with his huge horns the whole mountain on the side.

Now the bull again put the boy between the horns. They moved on and came to the sea. "Now we have to turn back!" Said the boy, "because no one can go over there!"

"Wait a minute," said the bull, "and hold on to my horns."

He bent his head to the water and soffit and sofficated the whole sea, so that they moved on dry feet as in a meadow.

Now they were soon at the Flammenburg. From afar, they were met with such a glow that the boy could not stand it anymore. "Stop!" He shouted to the bull, "no farther, or we'll have to burn." The bull, however, ran very close and poured the sea he had drunk into the flames, so that they soon extinguished and a more powerful one Smoke arose that darkened the whole sky. Then the twelve-headed dragon rushed out of the black clouds angrily.

"Now it's up to you!" Cried the bull to the boy, "make sure you knock all the heads off the monster!" He took all his strength, grasping the mighty sword in both hands, and giving the dragon one like that quick blow that blew all heads off. But now the monster struck and curled on the earth, causing her to tremble. The bull took the dragon's trunk on its horns and hurled it so high up to the clouds, until no trace of it was to be seen.

Then he spoke to the boy: "My service is now over. Now go to the castle, there you will find the princess and lead her home to her father! "With that he ran away to the sky meadow, and the boy did not see him again. He found the princess, and she was very glad that she was redeemed from the terrible dragon. They drove to their father, held a wedding, and it was a great joy throughout the kingdom.

13. A Sense of Being out Bird Watching

Steps for increasing effectiveness of the story:

1. What do you want to achieve from reading this?

2. Think about one thing you have achieved today.

3. Say to yourself "When I read this story then..."

Alternative introduction:

"As I read this and begin to drift comfortably asleep, I don't know whether I will find myself drifting asleep more to the sound of my voice or the words I read, or perhaps to the spaces between the words. And as I drift comfortably asleep I'll just read this story to myself."

So, as you listen to me, you can begin to drift comfortably asleep and while you begin to drift comfortably asleep you can allow yourself to get comfortable and allow your eyes to close. And I don't know whether you will drift off to sleep with the words that I use, with the sound of my voice, or perhaps with the spaces between my words.

And you can have a sense of being out bird watching one day. Of being in a little shed, a little bird watching shack, with some binoculars gazing out from this quiet spot. And you are gazing out through some woodland, over a large valley and you can see different birds in the nearby bits of woodland, but you can also see a large circling bird of prey in the distance in the valley and you can see it so gracefully circling. Seeming to use almost no effort and you look through binoculars at that graceful bird of prey and you have that unusual experience where, when you watch that through binoculars you shut off from the reality around you and awareness of the shack and awareness of everything else, to almost like you are very near to the bird, almost flying with them.

And while you watch that bird flying so gracefully and effortlessly, you begin to have a sense of thinking what it must be like to be able to fly like that, to be able to drift around in the sky, to rise up on warm air currents, circle round, to have the excellent vision of that bird. To see so clearly and so far and you can find yourself imagining that so strongly, that all of a sudden you become the bird. Seeing through the bird's eyes, flying drifting, soaring high in the sky, feeling weightless, floating, circling around, seeing woodland in the distance, seeing the vast expanse of the valley, green grass. Noticing bits of movement jump out at you as creatures scurry around on the ground. Seeing the way, the tops of the trees vibrate in the breeze and just feeling that sense of calmness, of peace and simplicity, at just flying and floating so gracefully with so little effort.

And while you continue to fly gracefully, you start exploring. And it is as if somehow you have taken over this bird. And a part of you is thinking 'Am I still in the shack watching the bird and somehow, I have drifted into a daydream, or was I watching the bird so intensely that I have got into the bird's psyche, somehow managed to get into the bird's mind?'. And either way, you go with the experience. You notice this fast-flowing river and you decide to soar down, fly over that water and you take some time to soar down and fly over the water, going in the direction the water is going, as it cascades down different waterfalls around rocks, through rapids and you fly just above the water, feeling the spray from the water, smelling the water, hearing the water, as it roars in rapids and then goes almost silent in calm areas. And you notice if you get just the right point above the water you can feel that you are flying on a cushion of air between the water and your wings. And so, you fly on that cushion of air and glide and float and follow that river all the way down to a lake. And as you reach the beginning of the lake you soar up into the air and circle around again and think of the fun you are having, as a bird flying, taking all of this in.

You feel a sense of elegance and grace and you continue exploring. And you are now in an area you have never been before. As a bird watcher you have been and watched birds before. You have even been down and walked through the valley, you have even walked and seen some of that river and the lake, but now you seem to have flown over an area you have never been before. An area of woodland, only you notice something about this woodland.

Your eyesight is so good that you notice subtleties, you notice that some trees are slightly higher up than others and you notice there is a certain pattern to these trees and intuitively something tells you it is worth going down there and investigating. So you fly down and you are too big to fit through the treetops in this area of the woodland, so you circle around and explore and conclude that you are going to have to land at the beginning of the woodland, but you don't know how well a bird of prey is going to be able to walk from the beginning of the woodland all the way into the woods, but you don't see an alternative, so you fly around and land at the beginning of the woodland and as you come in to land, you bring your wings back, you open them wide, slowing you right down, catching as much wind as possible, catching as much of that air as possible. And you put your feet out in front of you and you have an odd experience, that just as your feet touch the ground, you become yourself again and you find yourself stood before the woodland.

You are still trying to work out whether this is a dream and whether you have somehow gazed at that bird so intensely that you are now dreaming and having this experience and yet it feels very real and undream-like. And you think, if it was just a dream wouldn't you just wake up by just deciding this is a dream and deciding to just wake up and yet it doesn't seem like a dream or something you can wake up from. It's not something that bothers you, it is just a curiosity.

You walk into the woods, listening to the footsteps, listening to the different sounds in the woods, noticing how the light changes as you walk into the woods. And the woods are quite dense and you have to push through and work your way through. And as you push and work your way through the woods, you notice that there are some areas that seem to be a bit higher, areas that seem to be a bit lower, like the woods have built on top of something. But you don't know what and you keep pushing and pushing, until eventually there is an area that is a little bit clearer and you notice that the woods have overgrown over some kind of old building. And as you walk around and explore, you find that it seems to have grown over lots of old buildings.

You keep walking and keep exploring and all you keep finding is more and more buildings like this is a huge area of many buildings. Then you find a bit that looks like a normal bit of land, perhaps a normal outcrop of rock and you decide to go and explore it and you scratch through the plants that have covered it over and you notice that it is a wall of a building that has partially collapsed. And you follow this wall to see where it leads. It seems like you have found some kind of building that would have been near the centre of this lost city. Then as you keep exploring, you notice an indentation in the ground and you notice that this is where an entrance must have once been. So, you start clearing this entrance space and you find that just behind a bit of rubble is a tunnel heading downwards with some steps.

You walk in to the tunnel and as you do, somehow, oddly, your eyes adapt to be able to see in this tunnel, like somehow you have got some of the abilities of the wild animals in this area. You don't try to understand it because you are too busy thinking that it benefits what you want to achieve, you want to explore this area. So, you head down deeper into this building. And quite a way down you find a stone slab that you think is probably in front of an entrance to something. And you start pushing around on the stone slab and around on the wall around the stone slab and then somehow, you just take a step and the slab moves aside. And it grinds and moves aside, as you walk through and you find yourself in a vast chamber.

Within this vast chamber, you notice that there are scrolls all around the walls in diamond shaped spaces and there has got to be tens of thousands of scrolls in the spaces around the walls, perhaps like some lost civilisations' library. You manage to carefully open one of the scrolls and it is in a language you don't understand, so you put it back and you open another one and it is in the same language that you don't understand so you put it back and you suspect there is so much wisdom contained within these scrolls. And you see, right in the middle of the room is a pedestal with an open scroll and the scroll is being held open with a golden clasp at the top and the bottom and you stand in front of that scroll, you stand near the pedestal and you assume you aren't going to be able to read this one either and you gaze at this scroll and everything on it begins to change, almost like a mist passing across the scroll. And it is like the writing is rewriting itself and the scroll ends up being able to be read, it ends up readable and so you start reading this scroll and realise it is teaching you inner wisdom, it is teaching you something that will transform your life.

You read the scroll with fascination, with wonder, only vaguely aware of the impact it is going to have positively on you. And you read that this one also includes instructions saying that all the scrolls can be read when held on this pedestal by this golden clasp. So, you go and get another scroll, you place that on the pedestal and clasp it into place and you watch as the writing transforms, almost like mist and movement and changing of the text, to become readable. And you read that one and it is full of knowledge you never would have known, ancient knowledge, ancient wisdom. Then you get another scroll, putting that one back and notice that that scroll also contains ancient wisdom. And you wonder how long it would take to work your way through the thousands of scrolls full of ancient wisdom in this place. And you read another scroll and another scroll. Taking in and learning more ancient wisdom. Learning on an instinctive level. Learning that with a certain focus, you can become the animals, you can join the spirit of the animals and somehow you had stumbled across that focus and by stumbling across that focus, allowed you to stumble across this knowledge. And you read and learn and find this knowledge fascinating. And you realise it would take too long to learn all of this knowledge right now, you decide to continue exploring.

And so, you put the original scroll back in place on the pedestal and make sure all the other scrolls are put away in their places and you explore deeper and deeper into this space. And as you explore, so you discover a giant underground lake and on that lake is a boat and this lake is totally still and you feel it is so still that it is almost unnaturally still, but then, there is no breeze down here.

You get into the boat and row that boat to the other side of the lake and get out of the boat. And you can now see that the lake has ripples and you wonder how much those ripples will die down by the time you pass across that lake as you return. And you carry on exploring, wondering who created this whole underground space, where underneath this city there is a vast lake and why did they create it? And you see some statues and you see giant pearls and crystals in the walls and you notice how they appear to be glowing, as if maybe there was tubes of light coming in from above, lighting up the back of the pearls and crystals. And you find a chamber and on a shelf in that chamber is the most elegant item of clothing you have ever seen. So beautifully woven. Something handcrafted that you know would have taken years to make. And you know this shows the amount of skill these people had, even though you don't know who these people are.

Then you see a puzzle on the wall and you know there is no further to go in this chamber, but you think it is curious having a puzzle, so you try and solve the puzzle. And after a while moving things around, trying to work the puzzle out, suddenly you get the puzzle, something inside you clicks and makes it make sense to you and then a secret door opens. You go through the secret door, going deeper and deeper into this building. And you see a room so large that you can't see the other side of it. You can't see the side on the left or the side on the right, you don't know how the ceiling is being held up in a room this large. And you walk into the room and after a very, very long time of walking in a straight line so that you don't get lost, just following the markings on the ground, you find yourself at another pedestal, only on this pedestal is a bit confusing, you see a perfectly polished black pebble.

And so, you pick up that perfectly polished black pebble, you feel it in your fingers, you run it through your fingers, feel the smoothness of that pebble. You then see a note next to the pebble that says 'Take me.'.

And then you turn the note over and it says 'Put me in your shoe and lose me, when the time is right.".

And you think that this is unusual, but you take the pebble, you slide it into the side of your shoe, feeling it is a bit uncomfortable, but you slide it into the side of your shoe, you don't know why you followed these instructions but you feel these people must have a reason and you are curious what that reason may be and you know the only way to discover the reason is to follow along, so you put that pebble in your shoe. And you find your way, with a bit of a limp initially, out of that room and you start finding your way back through the building. After a while, you habituate to that pebble in your shoe and you stop noticing the pebble in your shoe and you know it is still there and you know that if you draw attention to it, you notice it again.

You continue to find your way out and then find your way into the woods. Then you work your way through the wood, back the way you came and when you exit the woods, you don't know how far it is to get back to where you came from. You know you are supposed to be birdwatching, but you don't know how to get back to where you are birdwatching. And then you feel this compulsion to jump. And you jump up in the air and instantly, you seem to have wings and you do a large flap and launch yourself higher into the air and you notice you are that bird again and you fly and you catch an updraft of warm air and you spiral round and rise up higher into the air. You don't give it any thought, you just seem to know your way back to where you were first seen as a bird and you fly your way back to that location and circle around in that location and the next minute you feel a slight curious feeling and realise you are looking through some binoculars at the bird and you wonder whether that was all a dream and are curious what it was all about. Then you look down and notice you have a pebble in your shoe and realise it wasn't all a dream. Something happened, some experience. And you don't know what it all means and you decide to follow those instructions of keeping that pebble in your shoe until such time as it is just naturally time to lose the pebble. And so that is what you decide to do.

14. The Adventurous Shark

Far out in the heart of the big blue sea, there lived a shark whose name was Ryan. Ryan was a beautiful blue shark, with a wide, big-toothed smile. He was also an excellent swimmer.

When Ryan was a baby shark, he loved swimming around the sea and exploring what lay in the water near their home. Every day, Ryan would wake up, and after having breakfast, he would wave goodbye to his mother with his little fins and dart outside their underwater cave to look for a new adventure.

Outside, he would be joined by his friends, Pago and Mia. They would first go around the neighborhood to see what's new, and then they would extend their forays into the nearby forest of seaweed and coral reefs. Every so often, a family would have new kids, and it was always fun to meet them and welcome them to the neighborhood. Pago was a little older, and Mia was a little younger than Ryan, but that was never a problem for them, and they always found many things that they liked in common. Sometimes, they would notice a new growth on a coral or a missing branch in the seaweed, and they would play guessing games on what might have happened to it.

"Maybe a sea cow ate it," Ryan would say.

"Or maybe someone made a nest with it," Mia would say.

"Or, or, or, maybe Miss Simone, the octopus, took it to sweep the floor with," Pago would say excitedly, then they would move to the next area to see what's new.

Sometimes, they would notice a pufferfish nest and go to marvel at it and try to count the circles and ridges.

"One, two, three, four, five," counted Mia. "Six, seven, eight, nine," continued Ryan.

"Ten!!" They all said in unison. "But what comes after ten?" Did they wonder? "Oh well, we'll be going to school soon, and we will learn everything there."

And so it came to be. They started school in the next season, and everything

was lovely. They liked their new schoolmates and made friends with most of them. There was a lot to learn, and the teachers were accommodating and kind, and Miss Tocci was even funny!

However, there was this one classmate named Rah. He did not seem to like the others very much, and he kept mostly to himself even during recess. Whenever anyone came close, he would swim away, and he hardly ever spoke in class. One day, Ryan approached him and said, in a friendly manner, "Hello Rah, how are you today?" but Rah did not answer him. He just turned away and continued to sulk.

When Ryan got home, and they were talking about how the day was, Ryan asked his parents why some people are sulky, and he related to them his short encounter with Rah earlier in the day.

"Maybe he is having a problem adjusting to the new school," said his mom.

"Or maybe he has a speech problem." said his dad. "You know, some people stutter or stammer, but it goes away with time and with practice," he added.

Ryan always marveled at how wise and insightful his parents were. "And what can I do to help him?" he asked.

"Just keep being his friend," answered his dad.

"And maybe try teaching him a new song, like the one we taught you when you were learning to swim and would sometimes be afraid. Do you remember it?" asked his mom.

"Oh, yes! I had forgotten about that song. Let's sing it, mama; remind me the words please," Ryan pleaded.

"Oh, alright," said his mom. But first, go get ready for bed, then I'll be with you shortly to sing the song.

"Yay!" said Ryan, and off he went to get ready for bed.

When his mom came in, Ryan was ready to start right away. "Okay, do you remember how we start?" Mom asked.

"Yes," replied Ryan. "Breathe in, and hold,

One, two, three, then breathe out "Good job!" said mom.

"Breathe in, and hold,

Four, five, six, whistle out," sang mom

"Yes, yes, I remember now!" cried Ryan. Then in unison, they sang. Breathe in, and hold,

Seven, eight, nine, flap your fins Breathe in, and hold,

Up to ten, let's return."

"Now, I remember it all," said Ryan, "Can we sing it one more time?" "Alright, dear; just this once, then it's bedtime," said his mom.

"Breathe in, and hold,

One, two, three, then breathe out Breathe in, and hold,

Four, five, six, whistle out Breathe in, and hold,

Seven, eight, nine, flap your fins Breathe in, and hold,

Up to ten, let's return."

"You two sound terrific." said dad. "But it's bedtime now, so goodnight, son," he said as he kissed Ryan goodnight. Dad and mom both went out. Ryan was glad to have remembered the breathing song and couldn't wait to teach it to Rah. He thought about the song lyrics again as he drifted off to sleep.

The next day was the beginning of a long weekend. As usual, Mia and Pago came around, and the trio went seeking adventure. They swam much further than they were used to, and Pago noticed that Ryan was quiet most of the way.

"Hey, Ryan, what's up, buddy? You are very quiet today."

"Oh, nothing," said Ryan as he swept a pebble aside with his fin, and they continued in silence. Mia, Ryan, and Pago did not realize how far they were from home until they tried to ascend and found that they were already deep inside a cavern. "What do we do now?" asked Mia with fear in her voice.

"Oh, my! I was so deep in thought about Rah that I did not even realize where we are!" shouted Ryan, who had just now snapped from his reverie.

"What about Rah? And what d-d-d-do we do now?" Asked Pago

"Oh, you know, how he's always quiet at school, in class, and at recess."

Just then, they heard a loud splashing from the darker part of the cave, moving swiftly toward them. The three turned and swam as fast as their little fins could carry them, but they were not fast enough. They heard growling and turned back to see what it was. A great white shark with pointy, gleaming teeth was coming toward them.

"What itty bitty little dudes! Go get them, bro!" He growled.

From the little light streaming into the cave, the youngsters saw a familiar figure swimming toward them. When he got closer, they saw it was Rah! He swam hesitatingly toward them but growled just like his brother. Taking advantage of his slower pace, they turned and fled out of the cave. They heard a loud, angry growl behind them, but they did not turn back, and neither did he come after them. For the rest of the weekend, the three friends played close to home and were a little apprehensive about going back to school when it restarted.

Come the next school day, Ryan, Mia, and Pago swam to school together and

kept close together all day, making sure to steer clear of Rah. They did the same on the following day. The school was no longer fun for them. They were always afraid that Rah would do something to scare them even more. Ryan was very unhappy with the situation, and he said to his friends, "Mia, Pago, let us try to do something about this. Maybe we can ask Rah why he behaved that way in the cave."

"Ummm, well, alright," they agreed half-heartedly.

At recess, they slowly swam toward where Rah was, and this time, he did not swim away or growl at them.

"Hello, Rah," They said timidly, but he did not answer.

"That day at the cave, you were very mean to us. Why?" asked Ryan.

Rah was silent for a while, then he told them that his big brother, Basa, was the bully in their neighborhood, and he wanted Rah to be just like him. He added that Basa had told him to have no other friend but him.

"Oh, how sad, said Ryan. "Here, I will teach you a song that my mom taught me; it helps me not to be afraid. Okay?"

"'Okay!" said Mia, who always liked songs. Ryan remembered then that he had not yet taught it to his friends.

"Pago, Rah, wanna learn it, too? "Sure," said Pago.

"Okay," said Rah.

Okay. It is called the breathing song. Breathe in, hold, and breath out. Now sing after me."

"Breathe in, and hold,

One, two, three, then breathe out Breathe in, and hold,

Four, five, six, whistle out Breathe in, and hold,

Seven, eight, nine, flap your fins Breathe in, and hold,

Up to ten, let's return."

Oh, it is such a good song! said Mia. "It makes me feel relaxed," added Pago.

"How about you, Rah?" asked Ryan. It's alright, I guess," said Rah.

Okay, let's sing it again. "Breathe in, and hold,

One, two, three, then breathe out Breathe in, and hold,

Four, five, six, whistle out Breathe in, and hold,

Seven, eight, nine, flap your fins Breathe in, and hold,

Up to ten, let's return."

"I actually do feel much better," said Rah.

The three friends looked at each other happily. "Told you, it works!" Said Ryan.

"Okay, fins in. Friends on three! One, two, three!"

"Friends!" they all shouted happily and went back to class, giggling.

After that, every day at recess, Rah joined them, and they always started and ended the recess with the breathing song. Sometimes, when Rah couldn't' sleep at night, too, he sang it to himself. One day, his brother, Basa, heard him and gruffly asked him, "What are you singing? Why are you singing?

"My friend at school taught me a breathing song. I sing it to relax and not to feel afraid," Rah replied. He was no longer afraid to stand up to his brother. Basa noticed this and was also perplexed that his little brother had friends at school. The tune for the breathing song, however, was so catchy, Basa asked Rah to teach it to him.

"Breathe in, and hold,

One, two, three, then breathe out Breathe in, and hold,

Four, five, six, whistle out Breathe in, and hold,

Seven, eight, nine, flap your fins Breathe in, and hold,

Up to ten, let's return."

At the very same time, Ryan was singing the same song with his parents at bedtime. He was no longer afraid or anxious, but he was glad that the song had brought joy to his friends, and especially Rah.

"Breathe in, and hold,

One, two, three, then breathe out Breathe in, and hold,

Four, five, six, whistle out Breathe in, and hold,

Seven, eight, nine, flap your fins Breathe in, and hold,

Up to ten, let's return."

15. Sitting at the Roulette Table

Byron had lost $400 sitting at the roulette table that night. He was sure that the remaining $200 in his pocket would go the same way, but he was determined to try everything he could to come home with some kind of win under his belt. He fiddled with the chips in his hand as the crowd dissipated around the table. In moments, a new crowd would form around him and the next round would begin.

"You wish to play another round, sir?" asked the croupier at the wheel. Byron nodded tentatively, not sure that he should, but being unwilling to relinquish his seat at the table, lest this be the round in which he would get lucky. He watched people as they milled through the casino, gathering around the table where he sat.

"Bet it all on black," came a whisper from behind Byron's left ear. His head whipped around, but he saw no one close enough to him to have whispered anything in his ear. Had he imagined that? Had he gone mad with desperation? He supposed it could be possible for such a thing to happen, but he admitted that he wished that it would have taken more than the paltry sum of $400 to send him over the edge.

"Just do it; you've got $200 left to lose and you don't even need that money. You planned on losing it, so either bet it all and get your money back or lose it and move on to something more interesting." Byron raised his eyebrows, considering the validity of the point made by the phantom voice.

"Ladies and gentlemen, place your bets."

"Got a number?" Byron grumbled, half for himself, half for the phantom whisperer, wherever it may have been.

Pardon me, boys, the whisper sang. Is that the Chattanooga choo-choo? Track—

"$200 on 29, black." Byron handed his chips to the croupier and folded his arms, watching the chips as they slid into the black slot for number 29. It took a fair amount of concentration from Byron not to start biting his fingernails in anticipation of the loss he feared. True enough, he didn't really need that money. It was part of a savings yield that he had intended to blow for entertainment, but some aspect of his gambling addiction needed him to win.

He felt, somewhere in his bones, that this win would be the thing that would keep him from spiraling into a habit that would eventually break him. If he won now, he could claim dominion over the addiction. He had danced with the devil and led. He had looked down the barrel of an addiction that ruins people and he had broken even in doing so. That addiction would no longer be an addiction, but a momentary venture that simply didn't lead him anywhere new.

"29, black!" The call snapped Byron out of his thoughtful repose. His eyes went from the croupier to the table in front of him. Chips were being pushed toward Byron and the incredulity was palpable.

"Looks like your luck is turning around, sir. Would you like to go another round?" The whisper hadn't left him, it seemed.

"Who are you?" Byron mumbled, taking care not to be noticed by the croupier or anyone else at the table. Talking to oneself in a casino could raise the eyebrows of people whose attention one definitely didn't want in that situation.

"Just a guy who likes seeing people win. You want the next number or not?"

"I mean, yeah. If you're offering, yeah."

"Okay, good. This next bet will take you up over the top on your winnings. Bet it all on black."

"Again?"

"Listen, man. I haven't lied to you yet. Bet it on 6."

"$400 on 6, black." Byron handed his chips back to the croupier.

The croupier dutifully took the chips and slid them into place on the felt grid between them. Moments passed as more gamblers placed their bets for the next round.

"6, black!" Byron collected his winnings and looked at his replenished pile of chips sitting on the cherry table in front of him.

"Now get up and go to the blackjack table."

"What? Why? I'm fine where I am."

"No, you're not. You're going to win three times in a row when you're still relatively low on cash and they'll get suspicious and kick you out. Now, if you rotate from table to table. You can win more times without attracting attention to yourself." Byron stood up and walked over to the blackjack table that was immediately adjacent to the roulette table. "Am I getting through to you at all?" The voice had become indignant.

"What? You said blackjack."

"I said don't call attention to yourself. You win twice at the table right next to the last one you were at, they're going to know. Go to the table over there, by the slots." Byron turned around and spotted a table across the room. He ambled over to it and sat down.

The voice guided him through winning at every table he went to. At some tables, he would bet it all. At most, however, he would bet only a portion. Going all in, the voice told him, made him look too sure of himself. Winning after going all in, it said, would just make them mad. Winning $600 in a round was acceptable. Winning $5,000 in a round was less so.

By the end of the night, Byron had won $12,000 and was feeling pretty great about himself. He knew that this was the point when tables would be speaking to one another, urging them to look out for him and to curb his betting and winning in whatever way they could.

"It's time to cash out, B."

"One more table."

"You heard me, big man. You've won enough tonight. You walked in here with $600 and you're walking out with twelve grand. You trying to tell me that's not enough?"

"I'm invincible with you on my side, aren't I? I can't help but win. I'll win one more time and then I'll call it a day. Deal?"

"I don't like this. They're going to peg you any second. You'd be better off just taking the money and running, pal."

"Relax. One more game of roulette." Byron sat back down at the table and handed the croupier all of his chips.

The croupier held the sum in his hands for a moment before placing the chips on the table. He looked back at Byron once the chips were situated and ready to be placed in their appropriate spot for his bet.

"What is your choice, sir?" Byron sat for a moment, waiting for the voice to pipe up.

"Hello? You still there? What's the number?" Byron knew that he looked really suspicious now, mumbling to himself before placing his bet on such a large sum. The croupier stared at him for a moment, then looked back at the mass of winnings before him.

"You know what," Byron said to the croupier. "I'm having second thoughts about betting it all. Can I just—" Byron held out his hands.

"I'm sorry, sir. Once chips have been placed on the table, we can't release them until the bet has been placed and the round has completed. Too much risk for funny business."

"Well, can I sit this round out and just get my chips back for the next round?" The croupier pursed his lips and shook his head.

"I'm sorry, sir. You'll just have to try your luck with a bet." The croupier was intensely suspicious of Byron, he realized. Had he not paused, had the amount not been so substantial, there would be no problem. The voice had been right. He raised the alarm by getting greedy and sloppy.

"I see. I'll bet it on 29, black." Byron folded his arms and stared at the wheel, hoping he could will it to give him the outcome he needed.

"21, red!" When the croupier announced the outcome, Byron felt a knot in the pit of his stomach. He had lost it all. $12,000 was gone in an instant.

Byron pursed his lips, knocked lightly on the cherry wood of the table before him and stood up to leave.

"Aw come on. You could have won that round. Put up another $200 and I'll tell you where to bet it. You can come back from that loss." The whisper returned and Byron's blood boiled.

"Where the hell were you five minutes ago? I lost everything because of you!" Byron was furiously whispering to himself as he headed for the door.

"No, no. B. You lost everything because of you. I wanted you to call it a night and cash out. You wanted to keep going and bet it all at the roulette table where you started. Did you see how panicked that little croupier was? Kid was going to lose his job because of you if you hadn't lost." Byron breathed in deeply.

The voice had made Byron angry with its analysis of the events, but he couldn't bring himself to conclude that the voice was wrong. If he had just followed what it said, he would have come out on top.

What was another $200? He could put that up with no issue. If he could turn that $200 into $12,000, he could be sure that he would listen to the voice when he told him it was time to call it quits, couldn't he? He could justify spending that $200 if he would get a return on that investment immediately. After all, it wasn't an addiction is all the bets were sure things, right? He wasn't addicted to gambling, he was just really good at it.

What he didn't know is that he had gone toe to toe with the addiction, just as he said he would. He danced with the devil, and the devil led.

16. Travel to Greece

It's vacation time! Sophie is ready to head out to the airport to travel to Greece with her good friend, Cara. But, she has to get there in time! Sophie's got to move quickly if she wants to make it to the airport and onto her flight on time to enjoy the vacation of her dreams, but everything seems to be working against her. Will she make it to the terminal on time?

It was a surprisingly drizzly day on that fine morning. The sky was overcast, swollen with the threat of rain ahead of what would be a busy day. The sun was completely obscured, and the darkened sky sort of lingered over everything. It was definitely not the bright, cheery day that it should have been, and it almost made everything seem a bit less exciting than she felt like it should have been. She was thrilled—in less than six hours, she would be on a plane headed to Greece—but she had to get there first, and it was looking like it would be a long day full of more than she expected.

Sophie sipped at her coffee as she looked out the window over her lawn. It was quite flat back there, with the occasional hole dug out by Bella, and without her trusty German shepherd running about, it felt almost empty out there. But, Bella had been left with Sophie's mother the night prior so she'd be supervised during the vacation. After all, Sophie had a feeling that if she had left the pup to her own devices all alone for a week, she would be returning to utter destruction throughout the entire house, and that was not something that she was really interested in dealing with at that point in time. Who had time to clean up all of the torn-up carpets that a bored dog would inevitably leave behind?

As Sophie finished up her last sips of coffee, she turned her attention to the list written on the purple sticky note sitting on her table. Along the lines, in bubbly letters, she had written her to-do list for the day:

- Pack carry-on bag
- Fill automatic plant waterers
- Make sure ALL lights are off
- Put passport in purse
- Lock door

It wasn't much of a long list, but all week long, she had forgotten to pick up her passport from her drawer. She kept forgetting all about it, and she knew that if she made it to the airport without her passport, all bets would be off. She'd let herself down, she'd miss her plane, and both she and Cara would be miserable. She couldn't do that to everyone! She really wanted to make sure that the entire vacation was as easy as possible to get through so they could have as much fun as possible. That meant making sure that everything on her end was as impeccably managed as it could be, and she was determined not to leave anything up to chance or fate—she was determined to make sure that everything about her trip was perfect.

It didn't take long for her to knock everything off her list, and that was with even remembering to slip her passport right into place in her purse as well, next to her phone and her keys. Just as she finished making sure that her purse had everything she needed all packed up, she heard a knock at the door before it opened up.

"Hell-oooo!" she heard cried out in a falsetto downstairs, and she grinned in response.

"I'm upstairs!" Sophie called back from her room, not even bothering to poke her head downstairs to see her friend downstairs. She closed up her purse and looked to the clothes that she had lined up on her bed. She had picked out a cute flowy skirt that hit her knees, made of ruffled material in a bright, floral yellow print. It was definitely on the side of bohemian casual, especially when paired with her white off-the-shoulder top. It was comfortable, breezy, and plenty flexible so she wouldn't be miserable as she sat on the plane. After all, from their local airport to Athens was roughly 13 hours, not counting loading, getting off the plane, getting through customs, or anything else. It was going to be exhausting—but hopefully worth it to have that time to unwind.

Cara poked her head into the door to Sophie's room and looked shocked at what she saw. "Sophie!!" she gasped in shock. "Surely you're not going like that, honey. That will... Not do. Not at all!" With a sigh, Cara stormed right into the room, shaking her head and tutting her disapproval. "Honey, how many times have I told you? No white after Labor Day!" She rushed into the room, her blonde hair bouncing behind her in perfectly groomed waves. Cara was, as she liked to refer to it, as a "connoisseur of fashion," and her wardrobe definitely screamed as such. Even today, she was wearing a strappy dress in black with geometric circles patterning across it in white. Around her waist was a thin black belt, tucking in and showing off her curves. Over her shoulders was a small, black blazer with ¾ sleeves. On her feet were two heeled, strappy sandals in shiny black leather, and she was walking around with a strappy black purse draped over her shoulder.

"What's wrong with white after Labor Day?" Sophie replied with a frown, looking down at the clothing hanging from her body. "I thought I looked great!"

"Yeah, maybe if you're just heading down the street for your morning coffee before you get ready for the day... You're going to ATHENS, BABY!! Dress the part!" With a dramatic flair of her arm, Cara tossed the bag onto the bed and immediately stepped into Sophie's walk-in closet, looking around for something. She rummaged around in the clothing, muttering to herself under her breath. Sophie rubbed the back of her head sheepishly as she waited around, catching only some of the quiet tirade that Cara was going on about. "No... No.... Not enough... Wrong..."

"You know, I think it'll be fine..." Sophie told her with a quick peek into the closet, but just as she put her head into the door to see what was going on, she had a bunch of clothing thrown right at her.

"No, it will not be fine! Be civilized, Sophie!" Cara tutted again as she walked out, looking at her handiwork that was currently draped over Sophie's face and shoulder. Cara had chosen out a casual dress made of navy fabric with a deep V cut down the neckline. It was held up by two straps over the shoulder, and the fabric had a pretty print of pale pink flowers growing across it. The dress was narrow at the waist and flared out toward the hemline, creating a bouncy swing to it when it was worn. "Wear this one!"

Sophie shrugged her shoulders. It really didn't matter that much to her, but if Cara cared, she'd deal with it anyway. She tugged her shirt and skirt and then put on the dress. The fabric was smooth as it gently clung to her waist and hugged in all the right places, and she loved the feeling. The shoes, white pumps, were pulled on with it, and she picked up her purse. "Fine, fine, ready?" she asked Cara, who clapped her hands and squealed in delight before heading down the stairs head of Sophie.

"I'll be waiting outside!"

Sophie nodded and looked out the window. It was still overcast and looked like rain would start at any point. Briefly, she wondered if what she was wearing would even be enough in the moment. Could she really wear that in the rain? "Well... I'll be inside most of the day. It'll be fine." She pulled her purse over her shoulder and ran down the stairs and out the door, locking the door behind her. She was ready!

Cara was already sitting outside in her shiny silver Prius, car running to warm up. The first drops of rain were beginning to fall. As Sophie dragged out her luggage and loaded it up in the trunk, she looked at the time—they had an hour to get to the airport and another two to get through customs and boarded onto their flight. Thankfully, their airport was only precisely 52 minutes away, according to GPS, and they'd be able to get there rather quickly—they'd just have to hope that traffic agreed with them.

With both of them in the car and ready to go, Cara was off. The rain picked up quickly as they went down the road, and Cara groaned. "We're going to be late..." she mused as she ran a hand through her hair and looked over her shoulder as she switched lanes on the interstate, dipping into the carpool lane in hopes of shaving off even a few minutes. Glancing at the clock, Sophie could see her doing mental math as she tried to calculate just how quickly above traffic speed she'd have to go if she wanted to get to the airport with any time to spare.

The rain was harder now, thudding against the roof of the car like drums as they drove. In the distance, they could hear a summer thunderstorm rumbling away, and occasionally, the sky, far from them, would flash for a moment. "What a day for a storm!" Sophie said as she looked out the window listlessly, chin resting on her hand and her other hand resting on her lap. She watched the rain drifting off the window absently as traffic slowed to a crawl. As the rain picked up, driving conditions continued to drop, and soon, it felt like it would be too dangerous to keep going at that rate. They had to slow down, or they would have been in an accident.

But then traffic fell to a standstill. Cara slammed her hand against the car's steering wheel. "We're going to be late!" she growled under her breath, leaning over to try to peer ahead of the car in front of her. Traffic was barely moving at all, and her GPS was reporting that there had been an accident not too far from where they were at that moment. "What are we going to do?" she lamented, glancing over at Sophie.

"Well..." Sophie began, deliberating over her words as she looked over at her friend. Cara looked incredibly stressed out at the moment—her eyes were wide, and her lips were tense. "We'll be okay. I'm sure they'll be able to clear the accident quickly, and we'll be on our way in no time."

"I hope you're right," Cara sighed as she slumped against her seat, letting her hands fall off the steering wheel. She turned up the music a bit, and gentle music played in the background, not really exciting enough to catch their attention, but it also made the car's silence just a bit more tolerable as the rain continued to pound, harder still this time.

"I am," Sophie said with a resolute nod, though the waver in her voice betrayed her nervousness. Still, she had to be strong—she had to be convincing enough for the both of them. Of course, she was not quite convinced anyhow—it was hard for her to believe that they would make it on time with the slowdown, especially when they heard the sirens approaching, and the ambulance and fire truck made their way past them to presumably where the accident had occurred. They could see the flashing lights ahead, so it must have been incredibly close to where they were. Had they left a few minutes earlier, they probably would have been caught in it. At the very least, she told herself, they were safe. They hadn't been hurt, and if the worst thing that happened to them was that they missed their flight and had to book the next one, then their days were still going better than the people who had been in that accident. Their inconvenience was better than the pain that would be felt in an accident.

Traffic slowly began to move, crawling through just one lane that they were able to merge into slowly. They crept along until they finally passed the wreckage. A red SUV's front was crumpled in, and the other car, a small silver sedan, was slammed into the concrete divider to the left of the freeway. EMTs were tending to people who were all sitting up, looking shaken up but ultimately, okay as they passed.

"Wow…" Cara breathed out as she glanced at the accident. She was uncharacteristically at a loss for words as she looked at the scene. It looked awful. Both cars were almost certainly a total loss.

"They're lucky…" Sophie whispered as she eyed the carnage. Aside from being shaken up, it looked like everyone was doing okay, especially since both ambulances that had passed them earlier were still there, doors open, with the paramedics doing rounds between the people. Both Sophie and Cara fell silent, radio still gently playing the music and rain still thundering on the roof.

The rest of the drive to the airport happened in relative silence with just the melodies coming from the speakers and the cadence of the rain rapping at the roof. Cara was driving notably more carefully as they made their way there, and though they were running a few minutes late, that scene seemed to give her pause when it came to rushing through the rain. It certainly was not the weather to be trying to speed across the street.

Before long, they made it to the airport and got parked. They were still two and a half hours before their flight would leave—giving them plenty of time to get through customs. They dragged along their luggage behind them as they walked through the rain, with Cara holding an umbrella precariously in one hand while trying to pull two-wheeled luggage containers behind her.

Entering the airport was the easy part. What came next, the constant waiting, was the worst of it. They had to wait in line to check-in, causing Cara to tap absently at the handle to her black luggage. Sophie tugged at a strand of hair, curling it around her hair as she people watched. There were all sorts of people out and about, and they were all going in a different direction. Some were dressed for sheer comfort, wearing sweats and a t-shirt while others were dressed for business, prim, and proper. It was interesting to see all of the different people going in, as well as seeing the people of all walks of life going out as well. Some of them were clearly foreigners, rubbing heads and speaking in different languages as they looked around in confusion and attempted to piece together English sentences just enough to get a cab while others were eagerly following their tour guides who seemed ready to take them to wherever they were planning to head first. There were some groups of young adults as well—likely college students heading out for spring vacation.

The people-watching was always Sophie's favorite part of being at an airport, and it helped her to pass the time. She'd imagine all of the different situations behind the different people. She'd start imagining whole lives for these people. She'd think about the people's vacation plans as they came into town. She imagined that they'd go to all the famous tourist sites in town—they'd go and see the restaurants and the beach as well. She assumed that they'd all have a grand time, looking over the city in their hotel rooms, or that they'd be spending time at a rental home.

Before long, she felt Cara tapping her back to the real world, snapping her out of her reverie. "Ready?" she asked Sophie, who blinked in surprise. She hadn't realized that she had been spending so much of her time just thinking about other things, and she nodded her head, pulling out her passport and letting the attendant see it.

Checking in and handing in the luggage was simple—then it was time to wait for boarding. They went through the security gates and stood in line at the boarding gate for their plane. The line was already quite long, and they still had another 30 minutes to boarding.

"Are you ready?" Sophie asked Cara as she fiddled with her purse strap, grinning at her friend.

"Oh, am I!" Cara echoed with a thumbs up. "I'm so ready!"

"Same! Greece, here we come!" Sophie was thrilled—she was so ready to go through the different sights they had to see. She wanted to see the ruins of Acropolis and get to eat all of the god food. She was thrilled about the beach that they'd get to go visit, and being able to go through it all on their own was something that was thrilling to her—she was so ready to be able to go through it all. Her dream as a child had always been to go to Greece, and she was finally living that chance.

Before long, the line to board was moving, and they were in their seats. They had first-class seats, at Cara's insistence. Once they were on the plane, they realized that it was absolutely worth it as well—the seats were massively luxurious, comfortable, and absolutely worth every cent that Cara had so generously paid.

The seatbelt light came on, and the voice of the flight attendant came on the overhead, informing everyone of the rules, regulations, and what to expect, and before they knew it, they were up in the air, high above the world beneath them and heading toward the open ocean.

Cara and Sophie toasted to each other with the complimentary glass of wine that they were each given. "To safe travels!" they said as their glasses clinked together. They both sipped and laughed at each other. It was going to be a long flight—but at least it was a flight in luxury!

17. A Different Dive

Jane plunged into the water, feeling the unwieldy weight of her diving equipment leave her instantly. The water lifted the burden from her back and, as she adjusted to the breathing apparatus, her attention was placed squarely on herself. Finally adjusting to the pressure, the shifting presence of the tank on her back, the pressure of her diving suit, and the pressure of the goggles on her face, she was able to look around at the stunning world around her. She could see the other divers from her group plunging into the water around her, taking pictures with their waterproof cameras, taking in the wildlife that skittered and flowed beneath and around them, and marveling at this whole world that lay beneath the island where they had been vacationing.

Jane floated for a moment, looking into the deepening expanse that lay before her. As she stared into the distance, she could see the shimmering blue of the ocean darkening toward the horizon. She didn't expect to be able to see so far ahead of her or that the water would look so calm from underneath the surface. She could see fish lazily ambling through the water, barely taking heed of, yet relying on the currents in it.

She made her way closer to the white sands that lay at the bottom of the ocean. The water wasn't terribly deep here, so she knew she could swim down to it without getting lost or putting herself out of her depth. In the white sand, she saw many small shells and sensed a movement that came from the current that danced above. As she watched the sands arrhythmically moving, she saw a small crab pop up from beneath the surface and scuttle under a nearby rock.

She gawked at the life that teemed around her, swimming from place to place and admiring its beauty. As she did so, she found herself drifting further and further away from the boat that had brought them to the diving site. They were told they could go pretty far away from the site, but to stay close enough that you could still see at least one other diver.

She made sure she could see one diver as she continued looking for more pretty sights to see under the waves. As she hovered in the water, she swore she saw something whip across the floor beneath her. Slightly alarmed, but trying to keep her breathing even, she looked around to see if she could find the thing that had slipped past her.

Over the occasional hiss of her breathing apparatus, she heard the gentle swish of quick motion through the water behind her. She whipped her head around, but still heard nothing. Out of a sense of fear and self-preservation, Jane made her way back over to the group. She stayed with them until the session was over and uneventfully made her way back up onto the boat.

In her hotel room, she couldn't help but think about the presence that whipped around her in the water. She really had seen it there, right? It hadn't been some figment brought about by the heat from being on the beach all morning before her dive, had it? Either way, she needed to get back to the water to figure out what it was.

She looked out at the ocean from the balcony of her hotel room. She could see the spot where they had been diving that day. It was dark out, so there wasn't much of anything to see in that spot. The waves on the water were choppier than they had been in the afternoon and the wind had kicked up slightly.

She felt compelled to watch that spot in the ocean as the wind blew and the waves rolled. She was unable to take her eyes off the spot where they had been that afternoon, and he had also been unable to figure out how she knew that was where they had been. She hadn't even needed to think about it; she just knew that was the spot. As she pondered this, eyes transfixed on that spot, she saw something glowing beneath the surface. Something... big.

She wanted to call the front desk and ask about the thing glowing in the ocean, but she couldn't bring herself to move from that spot. From the muscles in her forehead, all the way down to her pinky toes, she could not compel any muscle in her body to move even the slightest bit, as it would mean possibly interrupting her view of the brilliant light that blazed beneath the waves. She could swear, as she watched it, that it was getting brighter and larger at a pace that her eyes could barely process. It was slow but certain.

Her ears twitched as she watched the light. Was it... Singing? It sounded like a hum, a screech, a hymn, and a bell, all rolled into one song. It was not a cacophonous sound, though her mind seemed to insist that it ought to have been for all the elements that it contained. She was thankful that she couldn't will herself to move. Everything in her mind was screaming at her to jump over the railing of her balcony and into the ocean to see what was calling to her from the deep.

Before she could make heads or tails of all the things that were going on at that moment, everything went dark. The song, the ocean, the light, the room, the city below... Everything. All at once, the waves in the ocean completely subsided and settled into a calm, glassy surface that reflected the moon, which somehow also seemed muted. She felt the tension in her muscles release suddenly and before she could compensate, she tumbled to the floor, losing consciousness on the way down.

She awoke the next morning to the sun shining through the open balcony door, birds calling, and calm waves crashing periodically on the beach below. She was still on the floor, wearing her clothes from the evening before. She picked herself up off the floor and made herself take a shower, get some coffee, and get dressed. Once she had taken care of herself, she would get some answers about what had been going on the night before.

She entered the lobby and saw that it was business as usual for the guests and employees in the resort. People were milling about, asking questions about gratuities, breakfast, check-in times, and scheduled tours. She peered around to see if she found anyone that looked anywhere near as unsettled as she felt but there didn't seem to be anyone who fit that description.

She walked up to the concierge desk to talk to the sharply dressed woman there that wore a bright, happy smile.

"Excuse me," she started.

"Yes, madam; how can I be of service?"

"Do you know anything about the blackout that happened last night? What was it that caused it?"

"I'm sorry? Did you lose power in your room last night? I can ask the front desk if there were any interruptions they might know about."

"No, I mean the blackout in the whole… Did the city not lose power last night?"

"No, ma'am, I don't think there was anything like that here last night. Would you like me to ask the front desk?" Jane's mind was racing.

"Oh… No, that's okay. Thank you." Jane didn't wait for a response before she went back into the elevator and ran back up to her room. She changed into her swimsuit and ran back downstairs and out to the beach.

She asked about scuba tours that would be going back out to that spot, but the instructor said that there wouldn't be any tours that day due to a family emergency for the instructor. The man at the booth was simply there for equipment rental.

She rented the equipment she needed and suited up, heading right for the spot where she had been diving the day before. The spot where she had seen that impossibly large light. How had no one seen it? How had no one reported on anything that had happened the night before. Had she suffered some sort of heat exhaustion that made her imagine the entire thing? Maybe this solo vacation had been a mistake after all.

Once she was certain she had all her gear on properly, she dove into the water off the platform that jutted out into the water. She looked around for any sign of the presence that she had felt the day before. At first, there wasn't anything strange going on in the water around her. In the silent calm of the water, she began to feel silly. Maybe she had just chased a complete illusion all the way out here and maybe there never was anything strange in the water at all.

She turned around to make her way back toward the ladder that extended into the water from the platform off of which she had jumped. As she swam toward the ladder, she heard it. Her blood ran cold and she felt the hot tingle of alarm pulse through her body. She stopped swimming and listened for a moment. When she heard nothing further, she turned very slowly to look at what had made the noise.

Nothing. Before she could feel anything at all about the lack of a presence in the water with her, she saw it. Something barreling through the water from leagues away. It was impossibly swift, ignoring any resistance the water should have posed. As it dashed toward her, it kept its eyes fixed on her.

Her muscles once again refused to move in any measure as she met its eyes. Dear Lord, she thought. It's massive.

Its eyes seemed miles wide as its gaze held hers. In seconds, the monstrosity covered an incredible distance. Jane tried to brace herself for impact as it closed in, but she could only float, powerless. Its immense mouth opened as it got mere feet from her. Its teeth were jagged and craggy. Each one would have been deadly on its own if it had been wielded by a person. Lined into the gaping maw before her, they were the gateway to oblivion.

As the darkness enveloped her, she could swear that she heard humming… Humming that also seemed like a screech, a hymn, with just a hint of bells. My God, it's beautiful, she thought.

18. A Strange Day

There was a strange day last year when something inside me changed.

I was living normally.

Work was the same ball of stress that it had always been.

Every morning I would wake up to the same bowl of cereal and the same cold linoleum floor.

Wearing the same suit, I would commute to my office job, come home, rinse repeat.

I can almost pinpoint the moment that things began to shift.

My phone rang super early one morning.

I pounded it with my closed fist, believing that it was my alarm clock.

I am not capable of discerning sounds before eight a.m., apparently.

The device was sent careening beneath my bed, leaving me scrambling to both find and shut it up.

My boss had called to inform me that I would not be necessary at work for the next week.

I believe they were remodeling or repairing something on the floor which I worked.

I was salaried so they could have taken all the time they needed.

I was thrilled to be set free for a week.

My normal answer to having some time away from my job would have been to lay around all day watching terrible reality television.

There was a small voice in the back of my head ushering me to take a different approach this time.

It was almost as if my body were calling out for a peace that I didn't know I needed.

I had to dig through my closet to find attire that was not specifically designated for work.

While looking through my wardrobe, I noticed an old bathing suit.

It was at that moment that brilliance struck.

I would need to begin packing now.

The area I live in was only three hours from the coast.

It was just after noon when I found myself pulling into a parking lot that was directly attached to public beach access.

It had been so long since I had taken any sort of vacation and I had never done so alone. Something inside was crying out for stillness.

I grabbed a towel from the backseat of my car and changed into my flipflops.

I placed my phone inside the glove compartment.

This was going to be an experiment for me.

I would venture out onto the beach and just take in the moment, as it was occurring.

No distractions.

From the moment I opened the door to my vehicle, my nostrils were greeted with the brackish ocean air.

The scent brought with it a familiar and nostalgic ache.

I recalled the hazy days of my youth spent tossing in the waves beneath a radiant summer sun.

The ocean breeze is something that isn't replicated on any other occasion.

Sometimes a cool draft on a warm day will steal your mind away to moments spent seaside, but it is never quite the same.

It had called to me through my fondest memories.

I sat facing the rhythmically crashing waves as they broke upon the shore.

I took off my slides so that I could dig my toes into the sand; it molded like clay around my feet.

There was nothing to do except look at the beach and enjoy the beautiful blue sky.

Seagulls passed overhead, squawking intermittently.

The wind picked up every now and then, sending the occasional other beachgoers scrambling for their towels.

There was laughter emanating sparsely from either side of me.

Families had probably arrived to enjoy their time away from the daily grind.

I had never placed much value on vacations.

I was much more a "staycation" sort of man.

I was beginning to see the reason that people drove for so long to reach these places.

It feels stagnating to sit in the same environment all the time.

When I was allowed to have time off, all of my days seemed to run together.

They are all a short blur because of the way I just sat and watched the time pass.

I was beginning to open my eyes to the idea of exploring in my free time.

I had always admired people who took on adventures.

Could I potentially be one of those people?

I was feeling so motivated that I grabbed my towel and stood up.

I would walk along the shore rather than just sitting in place.

Sitting was an activity that the old me would love.

New me would have to investigate.

I began my march down the shoreline, which seemed to go on forever.

I tried to come up with a way to mark my starting point, but I was rather lacking landmarks.

I was just going to have to do my best to find my car later.

Time passed without my acknowledgment because my mind was busy soaking in this foreign scenery.

There were so many charming oceanfront houses.

These structures were painted the most eccentric colors.

Something about having a house near water must give the owners a creative license.

They were much more interesting than residences in my town.

I eventually wandered onto a boardwalk.

There were so many interesting shops and hole-in-the-wall restaurants.

I love the décor in seaside diners; I learned that day.

I also learned that I have an affinity for lobster rolls.

Every tiny store that I entered (save a couple of clothing places) looked as though it had been frozen in time a decade before.

There was a small tin building that looked a little dinged and rough around the edges.

Above the threshold, there was a huge neon sign that read Arcade.

I must have killed an hour inside this place.

It had the perfect ambiance.

The carpet was a faded maroon color with spots where it had suffered spills over the years.

The paint on the walls had chipped away some, exposing the grey beneath.

There picnic tables inside that had been written on in permanent marker by overzealous children.

To spite the arcade's flaws, the inside was aglow.

There were neon lights everywhere.

So many games that I hadn't played since childhood stood before me now, ready to accept my coins.

I was determined to reclaim my top score title from an alien video game that peaked in the nineties.

I collected my random assortment of prizes.

I left with a cheap frisbee, a sunset-colored bouncy ball and candy that I can only hope were manufactured sometime this year.

I was having a perfect day so far.

I was convinced that there was nothing left on the menu today that could top the joy I felt in this moment.

I journeyed all the way back to my car.

I was not tasked with finding a hotel.

Summer was not quite in full swing yet, so I was hopeful.

The place that I found was beautiful and quaint, right on the shore.

I settled in and then returned to the beach in time for sunset.

I sat in the sand and watched as the light played off of the ocean water and waves as they crashed into one another.

Brilliant colors unfolded across the horizon.

The gentle wind caressed my cheek and reminded me to be appreciative of myself for my decision to take this risk. As I stare at the beauty before me.

The salty air filled my lungs.

I imagined that the breaths that I was taking were healing me from the inside out.

Visualization Exercise

Sit somewhere comfortable and quiet.

Close your eyes and begin breathing deeply, in through your nose and out through your mouth.

Draw in your breath to the count of four and hold to the count of two.

Repeat this four times and allow yourself to sink into normal deep breathing.

Listen to the sounds and feelings of your own body as you pull in the air.

Allow your thoughts to melt from your mind.

You should feel the tension in your body begin to release.

Your muscles will feel relaxed and heavy.

The floor or bed that you are sitting on will sustain the entire weight of your body.

When you are feeling relaxed and calm, imagine that you are in a place where you feel comfortable.

It could be the beach, a field, a mountain setting, a desert, or anything else.

Allow your mind to be transported to this place for a while.

Engage your other senses in this scene.

Feel the air around you and the wind as it blows.

Smell the scents associated with the location that you have chosen.

Hear the crashing ocean waves or the rushing water of a river.

Mentally transport yourself to this place of peace.

Stay in this location for as long as you please.

Rest here for a while, away from the world.

Allow yourself to feel consumed by this environment.

When you have finished your time here, sit in silent contemplation for a moment before returning to your waking life.

19. The Adult Friendship

After another long day, Adrian sat on the couch with his wife, Bella. They both had busy lives, and having an eight-year-old child on top of it all made it even harder. Adrian was the general manager of a giant department store, Paris Goods. He spent almost all of his time at work, and it always seemed like by the time he got home, he only got to spend an hour or so with his daughter.

He also had a head full of thoughts that he wanted to share with people, but the only person he could really share them with was Bella. The game was about to come on, and Adrian told his wife about what was at stake today.

"Now that they have Brady, taking away their winning streak is going to be rough," Adrian said. He munched on cheese snacks as the game started.

Bella sighed. "You always go through this with me, Adrian. And I always tell you that I don't care about football," she said.

He finished chewing and swallowed his snack. "No one else is around to talk about it with," he said with a laugh, gesturing around the house. It was just the two of them alone downstairs with Avi in her room upstairs.

"When I talk about my TV dramas, I don't bother you with that," Bella said. "I have girlfriends I can do that with. You can surely find some buddies who want to talk about football with you."

Adrian stopped paying attention to the game and reflected back on his life. He didn't have any problems getting close to people in the earlier stages of his life. From elementary school through college, he always had friends to talk to about things like sports.

After graduating from college was the time things started to change. It didn't take long until he got married to Bella. For about ten years, they made their relationship their focus; by that point, the two of them weren't even sure if they wanted to have kids. Adrian was busy with his business degree, and Bella was busy teaching during the day. But after some time, they did decide to have a child, and Bella became pregnant with Avi.

These days, just a few things had changed. Adrian had become the General manager of Paris Goods, where he now spent nearly all of his time. When he wasn't there, he was at home spending time with his family. All he had to do was look back at the past twenty years to see why Adrian didn't have close friends he could talk to anymore.

He had people at work he was friendly with, but those weren't the kind of friends he needed. Adrian needed someone who he could let go around and say whatever he wanted with. Right now, the only person who fit that description was his wife, and it sounded like she didn't want to be the only person with that role.

He did have one place he could potentially meet people, though. The place he was thinking of was really his only option; At the department store, he talked to people on a daily basis. Adrian figured he was easier able to make friends in the past because he used to encounter the same people regularly. In fact, that was probably why anyone ever made friends. People rarely made friends on purpose; it just happened because they saw people often, and that naturally caused friendships to blossom.

The closest thing he had to that now was the people he saw regularly at work. He didn't exactly have any better ideas. What else was a grown adult supposed to do to make friends? He didn't think there were equivalent of dating websites for wanting to meet friends, and if there were, that wasn't how Adrian wanted to do it anyway. His best bet was learning how to be more friendly with the people in his workplace.

The main problem was, he was the boss. The risk of being too much of an authority figure to be seen as friend material was high, but he didn't see any way around it. He decided to do his best and see where it landed him.

The next day before going to work, he read the joke book he had on his shelf and tried to refresh his sense of humor. If he were to succeed in giving off a more casual aura, he had to learn some jokes. Then he grabbed his coffee thermos and drove to the mall. For the first time in a while, he was nervous about arriving.

Most of the time, Adrian spent nearly his entire day in his office. Continuing this old habit wouldn't help him get friends, though, so he didn't even put his work papers in there when he arrived. Instead, he would spend the day helping employees inside the store. They were certain to be surprised to find their boss walking through the store for the whole day, and he knew that. He did his best to be as unassuming and laid-back as possible.

Unfortunately, they took it to mean he was checking their performance. It took some time for Adrian to pick up on this. One of them had to ask outright if he was doing anything wrong before he realized it.

This was his first major hurdle in making friends. As long as people were put on edge just because he was around, he couldn't expect to make friends with any of them. Adrian didn't see himself as a tough boss. On the contrary, he thought he was low-maintenance as far as managers went. Unless someone explicitly broke important company policies, he didn't make a fuss about things. Everyone seemed to think of him that way, however. Why else would they be acting so strange just because he was in the store instead of his office?

The store even seemed quieter when he was there. When he worked in his office, he could hear a lot more chatter among the part-time and full-time workers. With him around, they weren't doing any of that. They all acted very seriously and professionally. But he didn't know how else he would get closer to anyone. They were treating him like a tyrannical king, staying a good distance away from him, and doing their best to not do anything to upset him.

Adrian tried one of the jokes he read that morning on the assistant manager, Martin.

"A Buddhist goes up to a hotdog stand," Adrian said. "And he says, 'Make me one with everything.'"

Martin smiled politely, but he didn't laugh, to his boss's disappointment. "So what are you doing out here today? Usually, you're busy with general manager stuff, and we only see you a couple of times a day. You can count on me to keep things running smoothly on the floor, you know," Martin said.

"I know I can," Adrian said.

He had the impression that everyone was thinking the same thing Martin was thinking. It seemed like no matter what he would do, people were not going to be able to look past him as a boss at this time when he was trying to get closer to people.

"I'm glad. I just wanted to make sure you didn't think we were slacking out here. If anything, we're doing better than ever. You know more about the numbers than I do, but more people seem to be coming in lately, with the holidays and everything."

Adrian had a thought that he would normally have kept to himself in the work environment. But then he thought to himself that he would never develop a friendship with someone here if he continued to keep all of his vulnerable thoughts to himself.

"Actually, I just wanted everyone here to see me as a person instead of just their boss," Adrian said. He didn't want to share everything he and Bella had talked about, but he had to be more open and vulnerable if anyone was going to want to be his friend. "You and I, we've been in this place for a while. I've been here for over ten years, and every single day, I spend most of my time here. I just felt like I wanted everyone to see me as more than just their boss. Otherwise, most of my life is being spent around people who only see me as a representative of the company."

Martin seemed understanding. Like Adrian, he was why hard-working and meticulous person, which was why he picked him for the assistant manager position ten years ago. Adrian figured he wanted to be the general manager one day, and he would probably have that chance soon. The rumors said the corporate opening for regional manager was opening up, which Adrian was more than qualified for. Everyone in the Paris Goods circle basically saw him as the only candidate who was really being considered.

"Look, boss-man. I know you a little better than anyone else around here does, and I also know what they think of you. I can tell you where you're misreading things," Martin said. "Since I go with you to corporate meetings and we have to work together more than you have to work with anyone else, I know that you aren't that serious. The joke you just told me isn't a great example, but you can let loose and be light-hearted. But the other people working here don't see that side of you. They think you're strict, and honestly, kind of a corporate shill."

Adrian couldn't believe it. No matter what the employees thought of him, he wasn't anything like Martin has described. He did enforce the rules — that was how he got to this place in his career. It was what he got paid to do. But anyone who thought he was strict just didn't know how things worked around here. He couldn't let the employees do whatever they wanted. He had to keep the place running, and sometimes that meant reprimanding and firing people.

At some level, he understood where they were coming from. If you didn't know him, seeing him as an uptight boss would be easy. All bosses had to be upright to some extent. They got picked for those roles because they had personalities that liked to follow the rules. But still, he had to take some responsibility for it. They would probably have seen him a little differently if he had acted a little more open and wasn't in his office all the time.

Then Adrian thought of an idea. He didn't think he was totally off-base for trying to make friends here; he saw the people here more than he saw anyone else, and if he tried to make friends in any other environment, he would have to completely start from the beginning with them.

The person he knew the best here was Martin, and he didn't really know him well enough to consider them friends. But besides his wife and some others from high school and college who he could only keep up with online, his employees were the people who he knew the best.

That meant trying to befriend these people was still his best chance; however, this work environment didn't lend itself well to everyone being more open with him. He would need to spend time with them in a more relaxed environment if he was going to build any friendships with them — and he had the perfect idea to make that happen.

"Martin, where do people around here go out to have fun?" Adrian asked.

Martin looked like he had no clue what Adrian was getting at. "There's not much around here. I'm getting pretty deep into my thirties, you know, I don't exactly keep up with that kind of thing anymore. But the people I know who do go out just go to the restaurants. The ones that are really popular right now are the ones with arcades."

And so Adrian decided on his course of action. He would ask corporate for the money for a company-sponsored event at one of these arcade restaurants. This way, he could spend time with the people he already knew, but without the issue of them seeing him as their boss in the work environment. Of course, there was still a chance they would see him this way even outside the building, but at least it was heading in the right direction.

He tried to get the money from the corporate office, but he ended up having to pay for it himself. But these days, Adrian was doing pretty well economically, so he landed on financing the thing himself. Bella was fine with this decision after he pointed out it was her telling him to make new friends that led him to do this in the first place.

The night of the company event, far more people showed up than he expected. He was worried a lot of people would think it would be boring and stay home, but luckily, the turnout exceeded his expectations. Almost everyone from work showed up to eat good food and play arcade games.

The other good news was that people didn't act as weird around him as they did before. He figured part of this was the drinks a lot of them were having, but even his colleagues who weren't drinking seemed to be more open with him.

An event like this wasn't without its problems, though. One employee of his, Abby, had too many beers and started causing problems. The staff almost asked her to leave, but Adrian promised them he would do something about it.

He hesitated to confront her about her behavior. She may have been making a lot of noise, but he didn't want to make everyone see him as the boss again by talking with her in public. He decided to speak with her outside and call her a taxi ride home.

While he waited with her for her ride, he realized something. He was very close to making a scene out of keeping Abby in control. He didn't think of it that way a few minutes ago, but when he stepped back and thought about it, that was exactly how it would have come across. That meant his problem wasn't only his employees seeing him as their boss; his problem was also that he saw himself that way, too.

He called it a company event, but the truth was, he paid for all of it. Yet he almost behaved like he was their boss. If he was going to make them see him as a full person and not just the general manager, he needed to adjust how he approached talking to them, too.

The more he talked to Abby, the more she seemed to calm down. She still seemed embarrassed about having to go home, so Adrian was glad he made it as inconspicuous as possible.

They got to talking about all kinds of things. When he talked to her, it made him even more aware of how disconnected he was from all the people he worked with. He didn't see them as mere employees on the inside, but he told himself he should have been doing a better job of making them feel like he cared about their lives. The conversation made him confront the fact that he basically knew nothing about Abby, or any of the other people who worked under him, for that matter.

Abby had a lot to say. The beers had something to do with it, but he knew her to be talkative in the workplace too, so that wasn't all of it.

The two of them didn't have much in common, but she was still interesting to him since their lives were so different. Abby had boyfriends from time to time, but she was usually single. If he had to guess, Adrian would have said she was around Martin's age, but he got married to his wife a couple of years back. Even though she was in the same age range as Martin, she wasn't married, didn't have kids, and didn't seem to want to move up in her career.

She told him she wanted to get married one day, but she wouldn't mind retiring single, either. Adrian couldn't relate to that choice, but he knew for a fact that she had a lot of friends, so talking with her was like learning what it would have been like if he hadn't gotten married, had kids, and focused on his career. Choosing to focus on these three things had certainly made his life different.

He decided to take the opportunity while they were having a friendly talk about life, and said they should be more open with each other at work. Abby seemed like the perfect person to form this new relationship with. Maybe she didn't go out of her way to chat with Adrian, but she didn't act intimidated around him like everyone else did, either.

She made fun of his unceasing professionalism more than anyone else. Up to now, that made him not care for her, but it turned out to make her an ideal candidate for a friend. She didn't have to be inebriated to see him as human. He figured it was because she was closer to his age than anyone else at work.

He had a minor concern that Bella wouldn't want him to befriend another woman, but when he talked it over with her, she said she wasn't concerned. In the conversation, she told him that she trusted him not to betray her. Besides, she met her at the arcade restaurant, and the two of them actually hit it off before Abby went belligerent. Abby even appreciated his jokes; he hadn't been able to test cut his jokes on her yet, because he had been discouraged by the negative feedback he got from everyone else.

He found out there was more to her than met the eye. Ever since she was seven-years-old, she played the violin, and she was a prodigy back in the day who won all sorts of awards. He found out her father died in an accident caused by an earthquake when she was a child, and she said it affected her to this day.

His wife may have said their friendship didn't bother her, but Adrian still tried to keep a distance.

It was incredible the things he learned about her by opening himself up. He always assumed she would be lazy and sedentary, but he found out she rode her bike to work when the weather was good enough. Seeing another opportunity, he asked her about biking, and she invited him to ride through the park with her.

Going to the park was a nice change of pace. First, he went to the arcade bar, and now he was riding his bike through the park. The paths had a lot more bumps than he expected, and when they were done, his hair was messier than it had been since he was fifteen years younger. There hadn't been many chances to get his hair messy ever since he had a family.

The difference in their life paths ended up driving a wedge through their friendship, unfortunately. At first, they drew them together because they had a lot to talk about.

She wanted to hang out more than he could. Adrian had a lot of commitments preventing him from spending time with Abby. When he wasn't working over fifty hours a week, he had to go to a piano recital for his daughter or go on a date with Bella. They went out together whenever they could, but it wasn't as frequent as he would have liked.

By contrast, Abby had all kinds of free time, so she wanted to do things together a lot more than he was able to. This was why Adrian wanted to develop a friendship with Martin. Maybe wouldn't have had as much to talk about since they both had boring, typical lives, but Martin at least could be understanding of his time limitations.

Adrian could tell that Abby was getting impatient with him, because half the time she wanted to exercise in the park or do something else, he wasn't able to. Martin's schedule was a bit more flexible than his since he didn't have kids yet, but at least he wouldn't be as impatient as Abby was.

In the same way the problem with Abby was his lack of free time, Adrian had a problem with Martin too. The only reason he made friends with Abby was that they hit it off when she drank too much at the restaurant. It happened naturally and completely by accident.

He couldn't just force the same thing to happen with him. It didn't help that friendship was a strange thing for men as well as for adults. He didn't feel like he had the guts to talk to Martin like a friend in the first place, and the social rules for making friends at this stage in life were no clearer than mud. He was sure he wasn't the only adult who grappled with the same problem.

When he finally had the slot of time open for it, Adrian went with Abby to get coffee one Saturday morning. She didn't act impatient about his lack of time as she seemed to be before; she explained that she was only joking around. They were able to laugh the whole thing off. Telling whether people were serious was a lot harder over a digital medium. They forgave each other and had a pleasant chat.

"These days, I've been wishing I had what you had," Abby said. She seemed to have said it out of the blue; she was almost in the middle of a sip when it came out of her mouth. "It feels like limbo. My life, I mean."

"Funny you say that because I would describe my life in the exact same way. Our friendship is the only new thing that has happened in a very long time," Adrian said.

The two of them had gotten much closer over the past months, and he found himself confessing this sort of thing recently. While this was his goal — to make friends — it hadn't turned out quite like he expected.

"At least you've gotten to a respectable place in life," Abby replied. "I don't care what people think about the way I live, but I do wish I had gone a more traditional route with mine recently."

The two of them had gotten much closer over the past months, and he found himself confessing this sort of thing recently. While this was his goal — to make friends — it hadn't turned out quite like he expected.

"We don't have to sit here and complain about what isn't going our way, though," Adrian said. "Maybe we can find a way to help each other. I know it's hard with my schedule and everything, but we can make it work. I can try to set you up with one of my old friends from college. Granted, it's been a long time since I've been able to talk with any of them in person, but it's a place to start."

Abby's face lit up like she had been waiting for him to say that. "I've actually been thinking of something similar to you. You've been saying you don't get as much excitement out of your life as you used to, but we can do something about that. The two of us can make a bucket list together, and I'll even help you with it."

Adrian's eyes widened. He may have said he wanted to do something more exciting, but he had no idea what kinds of things might be on this bucket list.

"To be honest, I'm a little nervous about what you have in mind. I did say I wanted more to freshen up this life of mine, and I guess there's not anything better I could really do except for try to do some items on a bucket list."

It was settled. Adrian took some time off work so he could do a few of the things on the bucket list Abby made for him. After talking it over with his wife, she agreed this was the next step in his journey, but she just asked him to do his best not to let it take over his life.

The first item on the list was bungee jumping. Abby went with him, and they both jumped off the edge of a bridge. The anticipation before the jump was a lot harder than the actual fall.

Abby returned to her ordinary life after bungee jumping with Adrian, but Adrian got a rush from it that he wasn't ready to leave behind.

He took the bucket list she made to heart and did as many of them as he could afford to with his limited time and money.

He went to both coasts of the country. While he was there, he took lessons to learn how to surf. He rode a mechanical bull. He went on a hot air balloon for the first time. He saw the Grand Canyon.

Adrian knew his wife wouldn't be happy with how much he spent on these excursions, but it was his money, and he didn't spend so much that they didn't have enough for the necessities.

He spent a bit over a month working on his bucket list. There were still things left on the list, but he knew he eventually had to return home. After taking his trip to the West Coast, he returned home to his family and job.

Bella was extremely unhappy with him. Facing her was something he had been dreading for the whole time he was gone.

"You were gone for weeks longer than you said. And when you finally get back, all you have for me are excuses for what kept you away," Bella said.

The two of them had fought before, but hearing the tone she was giving him now was extremely rare. If it hadn't been for the strong foundation they had built for their marriage of the past years, he wouldn't have been so confident that they would be able to stick it out. Still, seeing her get like this made him feel horrible about what he did.

"I'm sorry," was all he knew to say. He told her that he would do a better job of keeping her in the know, but she didn't accept that.

She told him he was not going to pursue any other items on that list until they sorted out their relationship.

With his obsession over having friends, Adrian had forgotten the most important friendship he had: the one with his wife. She forgave him but said he was on thin ice. He said he was going to make their friendship a priority before he went back to any of this bucket list stuff that he had started to try to mix things up.

Adrian had plenty of time to mend his relationship, too. When he got back to his office at work, he found out that he no longer had a job. He got into the store to see Martin doing the duties of a general manager. Of all people, Abby was the assistant manager.

Before he could worry too much, Martin promised him he had a connection to get him something new. It didn't pay as much as his old job, but the money would still be enough, and the position and company were both respectable enough. The job was as a manager at a competitor's store on the other end of the mall, and Adrian rushed to take advantage of Martin's connection. Martin wished him luck on this next stage of his life.

He had just wanted to break up the monotony in his life. But it by looking for novelty, he had left behind all the things he used to take for granted.

Looking at it another way, however, he didn't think it could have gone any other way. He would never have said it like that to Bella, but he didn't know if everything could have gone on exactly the same for very much longer.

He wasn't the only person who needed variety to keep life interesting. Even after he got all the things he had wanted in the long term, he still had more to want. They weren't the kinds of wants that made him feel empty inside without having them; in his view, all of those kinds of wants had been satisfied by his family and career. But he didn't think human beings were meant to be happy with whatever they had. They needed to have more to look towards in order to survive, and he was no different.

One Saturday afternoon, much like the first time they had done so, Adrian and Abby went to drink coffee together at the same café. They couldn't help but notice how their roles had swapped over such a short length of time.

She told Adrian to take his life one day at a time. The way she saw it, he should have been grateful that his wife was willing to forgive him over his abrupt decision to go on a personal trip to fulfill his bucket list. He knew she was right; not everyone would have been as forgiving as she was.

By the time he had gotten back in town, not much had changed in any other respect, but much had changed for Abby. She started dating Adrian's old friend Patrick around the time she went back to town after bungee jumping with him. Things moved fast and were already getting serious. When Adrian talked to her, he couldn't help but think she sounded like himself when they had first started being friends.

It hadn't even been that long ago, but it felt like it was. It felt like a long time because he hadn't done anything on his own since he had left home to go to college as a teenager. The odd thing was, back when he was a teenager, the life he had now was the life he clamored for. But now that he had all that he wanted back then, it seemed like there was no satisfying him anymore. Nothing was ever enough because of this human need to strive for more.

Abby may have taken a new role in his life, with her path becoming more and more like a typical one. But she still helped him talk through his own issues, and she helped him figure out how he was going to make everything up to Bella. She said it wouldn't be easy, but he was definitely going to have to do something nice for her.

And that was exactly what he did. He took out Bella to the most refined French restaurant downtown — a place that she said she always wanted to go, but they just didn't because Adrian didn't like French food. He would tough it out for her. He called a babysitter, made the reservation, and he surprised her by taking her thereafter, dropping Avi off.

Adrian still didn't care for the cuisine, but he couldn't get enough of the baguettes. Bella warned him that all the carbs were bad for him, but he laughed it off and let her have it.

It helped lighten the mood to have the technically good food on their table. Bella was easily the better cook of the two of them, but neither of them really excelled at it. That meant having fine food around was quite the rarity for them. He didn't know how she managed to talk as much as she did with all that she ate. She tried to explain that she didn't want him to eat fewer carbs from the baguettes because of health reasons, but because they would fill him up. He barely touched his own entree, so it didn't bother him, but he saw that she had been planning for her many servings from the very beginning. Bella made her way through seconds and then halfway through a plate of thirds before finally getting too full to eat any more.

"I'm not worried about the money, sweetie, " Bella said suddenly.

The whole time, he had thought she was simply enjoying her food. But the entire meal, she had been thinking through serious matters.

"We may not be as comfortable as we used to be, but with both of us working, and with how responsible we've been with our budget our whole life, there's not going to be any issues there. What did worry me was how unlike you, it was to go on these bucket list adventures without keeping up with me. Sure, you left a few voicemails a week to tell me you were safe, but it wasn't nearly enough. As far as I knew for all of those days I didn't hear anything from you, you could have been really hurt. You don't know what that would have done to me."

She dropped so much on him that he didn't know what to say. He decided he should stick to the basics.

"I don't have anything to say that will make up for what I did, but I'm sorry, and I'll do my best not to do anything that stupid ever again," Adrian said. He didn't say more than that — it would have come across like an argument.

The rest of their evening was pleasant and uneventful. He apologized many more times that night the way he should have done a long time ago, but there was no changing it now. All he could do now was try to make things right today.

Since things with Bella were mostly resolved, he thought he would try to finish what he had been trying to do from the very beginning.

With him not working at Paris Goods anymore, getting closer to his former employees was a lot easier. He still saw them at the same mall and chatted them up. Getting to know them was a lot easier without the barrier of the employer-employee relationship in their way.

It didn't take long until he planned a new event for them to meet up. He invited everyone from his old workplace, not just Abby and Martin. When the night came, even more people showed up than the first time. It seemed like people were much more willing to spend time with him when he wasn't there boss. He wondered if he could have achieved this kind of closeness with them if he had still been there boss. But it didn't matter anymore. What mattered now was that they did want to go to the arcade restaurant with him and everyone else.

This time, Abby didn't even have to drink too much and make a scene like she did last time for everyone to have a story to tell. In fact, with her new boyfriend there, it seemed like she changed her while personality quite a bit. Something about it didn't sit quite right with Adrian. He didn't want to tell her how to live her own life, but he took a moment in the night to make sure she was doing what she wanted to do.

"Don't you worry about me," Abby said calmly. She sounded like she was totally sure of herself. "I know it seems like I've changed a lot, but I promise you I'm exactly the same person inside. Now, the only difference is I have a new life to look forward to in the future."

"I hate to be that guy, but you did just meet Patrick. I'm sure you know what you're doing, but I can't help but want to make sure you're doing the right thing for yourself."

"I am sure," Abby said. "Things have changed a little. That's all. And hey, maybe he won't even be the one I end up with. No matter what happens, though, I'll have to thank him for showing me what I was looking for."

"What was that?"

"In short, what you have," Abby said. She looked like she was holding something back, and then she said it. "Adrian, I feel bad about what happened with your wife. With your going rogue and everything, traveling the country. I know that I'm the one who kind of pushed you in that direction, and I take responsibility for it."

He waved his hand in dismissal. "You don't have to take the blame for the stupid thing that I did. I own up to my own mistakes. Bella and I have talked about it. We went through it. At this point, we've been moved on from it for a while. No, things aren't exactly the same as they were before. But that's sort of how life works, so I'm not comparing. All we can do is take it day by day."

Abby nodded. "You're right. And even with the changes you've gone through, I'll always have you to thank as well as Patrick. We got the point of talking about you a long time ago," she said teasingly. "But you're the guy who set us up. So, thanks."

Adrian was shocked to see Martin go out of his way to find him and talk to him. They had talked many times before, but only if they were in the same place, because they happened to be in the same social situation. Sure, he came to the arcade bar with everyone, but a lot of people he knew were there. He could very well hate only been there because of that, and not because he considered him and Adrian friends.

"How's it going?" he asked Adrian.

"Good, and yourself?"

Martin shrugged. "Life seems to be happening a lot faster lately, don't you think?"

The two of them couldn't help but laugh. With Adrian losing his job and everyone talking about his midlife crisis so publicly, it was hard to do anything but laugh about it.

"I hope the whole management thing is going all right for you," Adrian said, and he really meant it.

"Well, it's not as easy as I thought it would be," he admitted. Adrian laughed again. Everyone used to make jokes about how easy it would be to do Adrian's job. Now that Martin was actually doing it, he knew from experience that there was no truth to the joke whatsoever. He never claimed it was the hardest job in the world, but there was nothing easy about doing the same monotonous paperwork every day while simultaneously Malone sure things got done that no one else knew about. This was a struggle that only managers could understand, and now Martin was a member of that club.

Adrian couldn't help but notice he was holding a beer in his hand. The Martin he knew never drank. He didn't want to draw attention to it directly, but he was curious about what the story was here.

Martin noticed him looking at the beer in his hand before he could say anything. "This? Let's just say I'm learning more and more every day about the struggles of making it through every day," he said. It didn't sound entirely negative, but there was a semi-serious tone in his voice he had never heard in Martin before.

The interesting thing was, he always saw the two of them as being very alike. But while Adrian was more on the boring and serious side, Martin brought in an aura of wit and light-heartedness.

He didn't think that part of Martin had totally disappeared, but he certainly appeared more like a serious adult than he had ever seen him before. He looked like he needed that beer to let go of whatever he went through today.

Adrian put his hand on Martin's shoulder. "I'm here if you need any advice."

Martin didn't say anything. He just nodded.

The two of them raised their bottles to a toast about getting older. Adrian didn't know if their friendship would last, just that they had one.

20. At the Bar

Every time Mark placed his hand against the bottle of beer, and he felt the coldness of it, something tingled in his being. From the back of his head, through his spine, and ending in the middle of his butt. That had been the only refreshing experience that he had known for the past three months since Lizzy left him. Shocked? Yeah, he was shocked that Lizzy could leave. Yet had he expected it. The warning signs had come, they were flashing in his eyes. At least he could not deny that one. She was unaffectionate, she could not be satisfied, and she increased the tempo of her nagging, hell, he could even say by a hundred percent. It was all just unexplainable, and he wished things would get better. Just like most stories like this, they never did. So, he just waited for what would unavoidably come, Lizzy, leaving him alone in the darkness that had consumed his soul with the prolonged times of strive and the likes. This is why there could be no other thing that he could rely on than on this fragile bottle, which he knew would one day send him crashing to the floor. Why he kept on to that too, no one could tell.

"When are you going to quit?" Clark asked him.

"I don't know, man. I just don't know," Mark replied.

That was the most real person he had still, but he walked away. Clark could not tell of any way he could have helped Mark. Any light that was truly going to set him at liberty would have to come from deep within himself.

"Help me, Lord," Mark muttered more often than ever.

On this evening, he had said the same words, while he yet turned to the green bottles at a bar. But on this evening, he could not deny, there had been a great restlessness over his being, all over. There was nothing he felt that he could do about it, but he knew the way to his favorite bar, and that was just where he went. If the universe ever did its work, or say, something like destiny, that must have been what was at work that evening. He met Tom, a lazy folk that walked into the bar. He had taken a couple of beers and seemed terrified. Frantic, he began searching all over for where his purse had been. He looked so much in panic, that Mark's attention, even in his depression had just been drawn to him. Mark was halfway through his drunkenness. At this stage, he could still comprehend to an extent of decent reasoning, but the speaking part was not so much what he could put up with.

"You little runt, you had better bring out my money or I am squeezing you till there is no life in you," the angry barman had said.

Why was he being so unfair? Could he not see that the little man had truly lost his wallet, and who knows what with it?

"I swear to you, man, I swear to you, I do not know where my wallet is. It was just here right now, right here with me. I swear it. I think I have been robbed!" Tom yelled, enough for every person who had been in that bar to hear him loud and clear.

"Every thief swears he is not a thief. I stole my wife's money last night. I swore on my mama's grave I had not even been at home at the time she speculated," a drunken man yelled from another side of the bar.

His comment was accompanied by the laughter of others. The barman did not seem to enjoy the rowdiness of the bar, but he had his eyes stuck to the little thief. Mark took his time to examine him for the first time. He seemed a teenage or a little above it. Say he was twenty-one or twenty-two.

"I can swear I have heard of this kind of trick before. You drink and you don't pay and you fake the loss of your wallet. Fucking loser. You are going to pay every dime or you will lose bones in your body tonight. I swear that to you," the barman said, sounding angrier. He had been a really big man, even he seemed larger than the regular size. At this point, he seemed to be advancing towards Mark, and there was no smile on his face.

"Leave him alone, I will pay," Mark said in his drunken tone.

"What?" the barman and Tom echoed together in unbelief.

"I will pay for the lad. Let him be. Add his bills to mine," Mark repeated, as he pushed a wad of cash towards the barman.

"Thank you, sir," Tom said, shyly, towards Mark.

"You're welcome," Mark mouthed at Tom.

"You lucky beast, now get out of my bar," the barman said, angrily.

As Tom tried to get himself together, preparing to scamper out of the bar, Mark spoke again.

"Nah! Let the lad stay with me. Let him drink as much as he wants to. The bill is on me," Mark said.

Tom looked at the barman and gave a sheepish smile. Furious, the barman slammed a rolled towel against the slab and walked away.

Tom, at this point, made fresh orders from the other barman and he sipped slowly and gracefully. There had been silence between them, in what seemed to be like through the entire bar. Tom passed cursory looks towards Mark and wished he could do something, or better still, say something to make him know that he was grateful for what he had done. Mark saved him the stress by speaking first.

"You did not have a wallet, did you?" Mark asked.

"Sir?" Tom pretended not to have heard the question.

"I did silly things like that as a kid too, you know." Mark continued.

"I am sorry sir, but sometimes, it just gets also crazy that a guy needs more beer than he can afford, you know?" Tom replied.

"Were those not the things that made us light enough to think we literally floated through life, being weighed down by nothing?" Mark asked.

Tom turned to examine Mark for a moment as though he could not believe the things that he was saying.

"Exactly sir, exactly," Tom finally replied.

They continued drinking and did so for a short while.

"You seem like the married kind, are you?" Tom asked.

"Is that a pleasant way of saying that I look stressed?" Mark asked, laughing.

"Perhaps," Tom replied.

"Well, I am not married," Mark said.

"Then what brings you here, why do you want to float?" Tom asked.

"Escape," Mark replied.

"What from, if I may ask?" Tom askes.

Tom went wordless for a short while. Meticulously, he took sips at his glass.

"Boy, I was once like you, you know, free and flying. Then I met this woman that I know I truly loved. Then things began to fly high for me," Mark began to explain.

He put his hand in the air, like a bird and he glided from the point of the table to higher and higher.

"Then all of a sudden, dash! I crash down like a little bird," Mark concluded.

"What struck you in the air, truly?" Tom asked.

"What do you mean? I just told you a woman I loved left me and that affected me so bad. What do you mean what struck me, kid?" Mark asked.

"Most times, we know what happens to us, but what we do not investigate is how we let what happened to us, really happen to us," Tom said.

Mark dropped his glass and looked into his eyes in unbelief.

"I swear, I have never heard a drunken man so wise," Mark said, laughing.

Tom burst out in laughter too and soon, they were both laughing out loud.

"Tell me though, what struck you. How did you give in?" Tom asked again.

"You know, it was obvious we were headed to that direction of things, but I kept hoping, holding on, something like that. You know. I kept wishing, even though I knew all was gone. Maybe that was not the crime," Mark replied.

"What was the real crime then?" Tom asked.

"Waiting to be loved, not knowing I had the power to love myself," Mark replied as he raised the glass again to his lips.

Tom gave no response to what he had said. He seemed melancholic, his face reddened after a while.

"What is wrong with you, man?" Mark asked.

"I remember when my mama died. Every single evening, for two months, I walked up to her grave to weep. I looked at the gravestone, looked at her picture in it and just cried. It was a festival of sorrow, every single day for sixty days or more," Tom explained.

"Oh, I am sorry about that," Mark replied.

"Then one day, I come to realize that I was drilling through the same sore that I hoped would heal. I discovered that deep down I did not want it to heal, I wanted to feel the pain over and over again. I thought that was the best way to keep alive her memory in me. I thought it was love, but I got to the realization that love was more. Love meant keeping ourselves strong too, and not feeling the worst for those we loved. Love meant letting go too. Then I chose to let go. It took a while, but I let go in the end," Tom explained.

Mark was silent.

"This is no philosophical shit, man. I mean it from the depth of my being, man. Let go. Walk by, walk past. That is life. We walk by things and people, if they are not meant to be with us, we must learn to walk past," Tom said.

"I hear you, kid," Mark replied, sober.

"Holding on to the blade that cut us would stitch no wound, man," Tom said.

In Mark's mind, he knew that it was true, everything that Tom said to him.

"I want you to go home, get yourself together, and be the best of you that you can be. All of this is for yourself. You have tried so long in being the best for others; you must put in the same energy for yourself now," Tom continued.

Mark thought about everything that Tom had said to him in that instance. He observed Tom as he hurriedly gulped down what was left of his beer mug, then he stood up to go.

"I have got to go, man," Tom said.

"But why, there is still much more to drink," Mark said, surprised.

"Perhaps. But I drink to enjoy and not to die. I have got no worries to drown," Tom said, patting Mark on the back as he walked away.

Mark wished after Tom had walked away, that he had gotten his phone number. Talking to someone of that kind.

Exercise

Begin by thinking of one particularly important person in your life and the relationship you have with them. Write down all the good qualities you like in this person.

- This exercise has to be interactive, you are allowed to consult.
- The exercise should not run beyond 20 minutes.

21. An Incredible Trip

Before we begin this journey downwards into the deepest realms of our sub-conscious, let us take a minute to physically and mentally and spiritually acclimate ourselves into being with awareness of our inner-sanctum, our internal workings. We will begin by going to a place of comfort, ideally a bed, or a very comfortable reclining chair, and we will relax our bodies to the furthest extent possible. Now, close your eyes, staying firmly on your back, with your arms relaxed at your sides and your legs rested downwards. Take one deep breath in, through your nostrils, counting slowly to four, and one deep breath out, through your nostrils again, counting slowly to four. Breathe in the breath of the spirit and breathe out the stress of the day. Now is the time to rest. Become aware of nothing but the air flowing through your nostrils, envision a steady flowing stream, smooth inhalations and exhalations, your body become weightier and more relaxed with each passing cycle of breath. Allow your thoughts to become completely still, as you focus on your core, your solar plexus, allowing your thoughts to flow outwards past your vision until they escape your being, while only holding and retaining the pure awareness of spirit, the holy serenity of the mind and body. Breathe in, one, two, three, four, then breathe out, one, two, three, four, each breath becoming slower. One... two... three... four... One... two... three... four... One... two... three... four... One... two... three... four... One... two... three... four... One... two... three... four... Continue this pattern of breath, expanding, and sink down deeper into yourself, becoming a voyeur of your own still, relaxed body, lost in time. Become lost in this experience as you journey further into the trance, and prepare for the road we are about to embark upon. Draw further and further away from your still, lying body, and into the realm of imagination, where images grow, the land of dreams that you are about to become one with. Erase your mind of all that is within it currently, and prepare the landscape for a new and fresh experience, in the farther reaches of reality. One... two... three... four... inhale... One... two... three... four... exhale... One... two... three... four... inhale... One... two... three... four... exhale... Now, with your mind, body, and spirit rested totally, entranced, and fertile, let us begin.

You are the sun. The galaxy is orbiting around you. You watch as they rotate and spin, and travel in shifting circles around where you stand, intersecting each other by what seems like fractions of an inch, an intricate dance around you. You hold out your hand, and hold it over a big, blue planet that echoes a warm, loving moisture. Tiny pieces of rock hover around it. The orb tingles your hands, and you feel a dearth of electricity course from it and into you and back into it. You are totally electric. You begin to move, floating, walking, out past the galaxy, and you realize that these galaxies are mirror images of each other, repeated over and over, tiny fractals, as far as you can see. You dance from one galaxy to the next, and with each transition you feel a new magnetic pull dancing around you, tiny energies, barely affecting you as you traverse this plane. This miniature, ornate landscape of suns, and moons, and stars, all dancing around each other, these quaint little machines, existing like a trillion little raindrops trickling down through eternity. Beyond you, even beyond all these galaxies, is the universe, what feels to be several lengths of the arm away from you are giant globes of energy, planets that dwarf the sun. You hover around them, and, as you do, you grow to their size, and the previous galaxies you had been born from shrink down to a level at which they are no longer visible. You are flying through space at an imperceptible rate, getting bigger, and bigger, and you know that no matter how large you grow, how exponential the growth is from the size you are now, you will still be nothing to existence but an imperceptible dot, the cage of reality so infinitely large that its barriers cannot be touched by a lifetime of growing at the fastest rate imaginable. You take control of your situation and start flying, like a rocket, hovering past increasingly large galaxies that begin to whiz by you in a great blur. Whereas they used to be identical but perceptible as individual units, now, at this speed, they really become one, and all there is can be summed up as one vibrating, holographic image, akin to frames on a reel of film, projected by at hundreds per second. You begin to wonder if you are still, the universe whizzing by you, or if you really are moving, as you feel that you are, as you told yourself to. Space is illusory. You are stagnant, and floating, and infinite, but always moving, and growing, becoming more. You come upon a gigantic star, many, many times larger than you, and its heat glows gold in a way that doesn't affect your physiology, but only your soul. You are aware that your temperature is at a homeostatic point, independent of anything around you. You are the warmth of your soul, and these are mere physical bodies. The golden glow, however, itself, is on your level. This is affecting you. The golden glow inspires you take it with you. You absorb the golden light of this sun and grow to dwarf the sun, with a glow that dwarfs its own origin. You are now the golden light spreading through the cosmos, unconsciously, merely an experience perpetuating through infinity at a rate that increases in relation to its own size; always growing, faster and faster, spreading, farther and farther, bigger and farther tenfold with each step. There are many black holes, bigger and smaller, and tiny pieces of you are sucked in, and spat out, all across the infinite cosmos. Each piece that is torn asunder is still communicating back to the whole, and with each new individual journey of the part is that much more growth given back to the entire unit. New clouds of gold are spreading, but they are all of a whole, all the same, all right there with you. They grow, and they meet, then they separate and spread, and all the while it is still smaller than a pinprick on the fabric of reality as a whole. This could continue for several infinities and still not make a dent. But it is so large, and so powerful; it is beyond the scope of man, to even perceive such a thing. This is every lifetime of every human that has ever existed, to the power of itself, squared, cubed, to the power of a variable that increases with each step. You have made yourself the source of infinite life in the universe, in the image of whatever came before you, the thing that you have become. It is unknowing, because to know itself would be a waste of time, as it is what it is, and growing, and eternal, and, more than eternal, infinite, to infinite degrees. Rolling past faster than the speed of light, but from a vantage point of such greatness it appears to be a drop of water slowing making its way down a sheet of glass, like a raindrop splattered on a car window. The light reflected off this stream of water houses within it mirror infinites that exist fractured within this one. Many lifetimes, housed inside each other, like the tip of a pyramid bleeding down forever with no tangible base, only ethereal and infinite growth. As we fly through space, we become larger and larger, and the distance between our molecules grows exponentially, making it so that at one moment in our lives we may be a trillion times bigger than we were at a moment previous, yet this growth would be imperceptible to the senses because all the senses, as well, are growing with it. Likewise, you begin to wonder how much you have actually grown on your journey through space, in dreams, if it is even quantifiable how much larger you are now than when you started. The swirling, dancing lights around you, that shift around each other as you change your perspective to almost become an infinite, solid wall, made up of tiny dots yet so thoroughly blended and so indistinguishable in their tiny distance apart that it may as well be one singular, shining force, they are all that is. As you have strived for the spread the golden light, the golden light has manifested across the entire solar system as it can be known to you, and while it is still spreading, and will spread forever, you have made a home of it, here, now, and you vibrate in ecstasy, a light within light, indefinable, save for the golden glow that is. You stop, for once, you rest, and you are nothing but the golden light. Forever, all that is, is here, now, completely still, yet growing, imperceptibly, infinitely, flying through space at the speed of light, stagnant, unchanging, for eternity and eternity after that, as you sleep.

22. In the Favorite Diner

Jack grabbed a jacket and an umbrella from his closet. He had thought of driving, but the rain wasn't coming down that hard. He was going to meet an old friend, in their favorite diner. He had not seen Carlos in close to a year.

The pair were inseparable as children. He could still remember the night they met. The fair was in town, and the smell of fried foods permeated the air around Jack. He was only ten, but he was already beginning to find his rebellious spirit. He wanted to ride all the "upside-down" attractions. His parents refused his requests, but he had worn them down enough to allow him to ride The Whisk.

The Whisk was a large metal abomination that jerked its passengers around, from one side to another. The seats allowed for two riders in each cab, but Jack was in a new town and he knew no one, so he sat alone. The ride appeared to be starting, but Jack could not fasten his seatbelt.

The ride operator was walking around with another young man. Jack did not hear the man saying anything, because he was on the other side of the attraction. He had apparently asked if anyone would be willing to take another passenger in their cab, as the boy was the odd number in his group.

Jack had enthusiastically raised his hand, in an effort to summon the operator's attention. The man thought that he was volunteering to take the extra boy, with an embarrassing enthusiasm. Thus, Carlos was seated next to Jack and the two began a life-long friendship. A friendship that just happened to begin with Carlos thinking that Jack was insane. Jack laughed to himself at the memory, trying not to cringe. His luck had always been a little weird. He opened the door from his building to the outside world. The rain had picked up quite a bit. He opened the umbrella and decided to take his chances anyway. Jack walked along the sidewalk, listening to the rhythmic tapping of the raindrops against the slippery fabric that protected him from the elements. He accidentally bumped into another pedestrian, apologizing profusely.

The restaurant was a tiny hole-in-the-wall sort of establishment. He and Carlos would eat lunch there almost every day when they were in college. The meatball hoagie was the stuff of miracles; he had never found a better tasting sub. Jack turned the corner to see that familiar aged brick exterior. There was a neon sign hanging in one window that said only "Hal's". He wondered for a moment, what sort of person Hal was. How had he never met Hal?

He opened the door to the diner, shaking off his umbrella outside before surrendering himself to the warmth of the building. Jack brushed his against the matt that lay in front of the threshold. A man behind the long wooden bar acknowledged him as sat down in a booth by the wall. Jack had missed this place. It smelled like grease and old wood, which doesn't sound nearly as pleasant as the scent actually was. He imaged that the atmosphere had not changed since the moment the diner was conceived and that he what he loved about the establishment.

There were tin photos of old actors and branded ads, adorning the wood-paneled walls. An old bulletin board in the corner held pictures of every regular. Hal's even had the classic framed dollar, supposedly the first to be exchanged at the restaurant.

There were only two lights in the dining area, and they were both hanging from the ceiling, attached to fans. This meant that the overall atmosphere was dimly lit and antiquated. He pulled the laminated menu from behind a metal napkin holder, flipping it over to find the hoagie.

To Jack's surprise, the menu had changed. Nothing looked the same. They seemed to have the basic fare, like burgers and hotdogs. There were no more subs and no hoagies.

The young man was not the sort to get worked up over trivial things, but he felt an aching in his heart. He had been remembering his past all day, with a heavy soul. Jack had let his friendship with Carlos drift away from him when his friend had moved. The missing hoagie was just enough to remind him how much had changed about his life.

Jack took a deep breath to calm his hurting spirit. He was not going to allow himself to be taken over by a single moment, especially not when he was about to see his friend. He used the other patrons in the diner to distract himself. At the table to the front of his own, sat a mother and her young son. He could only see a portion of the child's head, but he was immediately reminded of his youth. He had to stop remembering for just a few moments!

Jack watched an old man walking through the door with a smile upon his weathered face. He waved to the man behind the bar and took a seat in front of him. He could hear the men laughing to one another. Jack had become so engrossed in their conversation that he had neglected to watch the door. Carlos placed his hand upon Jack's shoulder. Jack hadn't seen him in so long, he could have wept. He stood up and embraced his old friend, whose jacket smelled of wet leather.

A waitress approached the table as Carlos found his seat. They both ordered a soda, Jack suspected that was because that's what they had always done. He looked his friend over. Time was such a strange beast. They were both still young, but so much had changed about their lives and their faces. Carlos looked tired, with pronounced shadows beneath his eyes. He had always been handsome but in an unusual way. His face was wide, and his cheeks were full. Jack had missed the glasses! He had almost forgotten about those thick-rimmed glasses. Carlos placed both hands upon the table and looked enthusiastically at his oldest friend.

"It has been too long. How have you been? You must tell me everything," said Carlos.

"I will, of course. What about you, though? How is your practice? Your wife?" Jack asked.

"I actually wanted to talk to you about that! There is something that I must tell you," Carlos said. He took his drink from the waitress. They told her that they would need a few moments before ordered and then they patiently waited for her to return to her place behind the bar.

"Tell me," said Jack.

"So, do you remember all those days in college? We would get lunch here almost every day," he said. Carlos ran his finger along with the chipped vinyl that covered the old tables. One of those tables should still carry an autograph from each of them.

"I do remember. I was just thinking about those days and how cruel time is. I miss having friends. I miss seeing you and all the dumb jokes that we would tell," said Jack.

"Well, miss no longer! I am returning to the city with Tracy. We are going to build our lives here. You and I will share so many new stupid memories and this is the last time that you will ever be nice to me. Don't think I don't remember who you really are," said Carlos, laughing. Jack felt his heart drop. New memories? This was the best news that he had heard in a long time. He had been lamenting his glory days so much, lately. He had completely forgotten that it was possible to make new memories.

"What? That is amazing! That is perfect!" Exclaimed Jack.

"Weird how this place never changes, huh? I think I may get the meatball hoagie, just for old-time's sake."

Exercise

Soundscapes

TIME TO READ: 2 MINUTES

TIME TO DO: 8 MINUTES

This exercise will teach you how to focus your attention, how to harness it, and how to maintain it. Humans have an amazing capacity for focus, but that doesn't mean it comes naturally. That's why we need to train our attention to stay where we want it to for as long as we need it.

In this exercise, you are going to focus on one simple thing: sound. What do you hear around you? If you focus, you'll probably find that different sounds are going on all around you: indoor sounds, outdoor sounds, even the sounds inside your own body, like heartbeats and breaths and your stomach growling. In this activity, we are going to learn how to keep our attention focused on those sounds and not let it wander.

1. Sit comfortably in a chair with your feet placed firmly on the ground, or sit on the floor with your legs in Half Lotus (crisscrossed legs) position. Rest your hands on your knees or in your lap. Set your timer for 8 minutes.

2. Begin by focusing your attention on the sound of your breath flowing in and out. Start noticing other sounds around you. Let the various sounds arise, then be replaced by the next sound you notice.

3. Continue focusing only on sound. When your attention wanders, notice this, too, and gently bring it back to sound. Continue the exercise until your timer completes.

23. Trip to Barcelona

During this trip to Barcelona, I want to treat myself to a front-row seat at a Flamenco dancer's performance. I've heard amazing stories of passion, emotion, and the energy of their art form, and want to experience it for myself.

To begin my evening, I start in the early afternoon on an outdoor patio with some tapas and two glasses of vermut, the unofficial beverage of Barcelona. The small bites are delicious and make excellent use of the region's offerings of fresh seafood and the most perfectly ripe tomatoes I've ever enjoyed. Vermut is an inexpensive yet delectable wine. It is enhanced with cinnamon and cloves, and I pick up hints of chamomile and rose. It warms me, and I leave the street pub with my appetite primed as I hear toward the gothic quarter for a slow walk to my show.

In the oldest part of the city, the sun begins to set the fading light casts long and interesting shadows across the landmarks. I remind myself to keep moving, to not get drawn in by the texture and the details of every new building I pass by in this labyrinth. Most of these streets are closed off to traffic, and I am free to roam as I wish, zigzagging from one magnetic feature to the next. Through one narrow road, I pass under a footbridge high above my head. It is decorated with details, the masonry of the arch at its base, and the latticework under the railings. The piece that genuinely catches my eye is the lace-like stonework that floats between the columns and arches along the top. I stop and marvel at how it was possible to create such a delicate work of art out of something as unyielding as stone. I sense I am not the only viewer and notice a couple has stopped and joined me in admiration of the architecture. "Beautiful, isn't it?" the woman remarks, to which he replies, "not as beautiful you, my love." They share a tight embrace and carry on with their sunset tour of the gothic quarter.

My walk carries me to the doorstep of the Barcelona Cathedral, the home of the Archbishop of Barcelona, Catalonia, Spain. It was on a previous trip that I discovered the long, rich history of the Catalonian people and their lifelong fight for the right to be an autonomous province. One of only four in Europe that lasted throughout the ages. It is an honor the people of Barcelona do not take lightly. This cathedral is dedicated to a patron saint of Barcelona, a young woman who suffered martyrdom at the hands of the Romans. The cathedral built in her honor soars over the old city, and its pointed spires still gleam with the last rays of sun sinking into the Mediterranean. The nested archway pointed bell towers, and dozens of gargoyles that dot each available point create a castle-like resting place for the spirit of the young woman.

I reach the hall of the Flamenco performance and hear the musicians from inside, easing the audience into the ambiance with the harmony of four guitars, the gentle drumming of Cajon, and the unmistakable clacking of castanets. The soothing strum of classical Spanish guitar draws me in, and I find my seat at the front of the stage just as the lights dim to signify the beginning of the dance. The music slows, a tall woman in a long, ruffled black dress emerges from behind a curtain. She walks to the middle of the stage; her look is serious. Her stride is purposeful, and at center stage, she assertively stomps both feet. She turns to the musicians, raises her arms slowly and delicately above her head in a fluid motion, a dance of their own. The entire room holds their breath in anticipation. In a flurry of movement, melody, and a touch of madness, the musicians strike up their song. The dancer claps along in a feverish rhythm and tells a story through her body. I am entranced by her power and elegance, the speed and precision that she maneuvers her feet, and hands and emotions in time with the music. She directs the musicians, challenging them to keep up with her creativity. She is the matador and the musicians her bull, her body is the cape, and they are all entwined in the organic masterpiece of Flamenco dance. I lose myself entirely in the moment as each enters and exits the stage, each with a story to dance and a passion for sharing. An hour after the first chord is strung, I find myself in a standing ovation, clapping vigorously with the rest of the audience in total awe of what we collectively witnessed.

The show is over, and audience members pour out of the hall and into the dark streets of Barcelona. As I walk, I try to mimic the skill of the dancers expressing themselves in dance. I gain an immediate appreciation for just how challenging the art form is. I hear laughter behind me and turn to see I am not the only traveler to make an attempt. We share a smile about our shared clumsiness, and I begin to walk back to the hotel. I pass by a small restaurant, with its table still out on the patio, and I recognize the couple from our bridge earlier in the evening. She is sitting on his lap, and they share a delicious looking dessert, he feeds her a bite, but it falls onto her skirt, they laugh. I hope they jump up and perform a dance to illustrate their innocent and passionate love for each other right there in the street.

Exercise

Feeling Identification

Exercise time: 10 minutes

Benefit: Identifies and expresses feelings

MATERIALS: Paint pens, crayons, or markers (whichever you prefer); 1 sheet of 18-by-24-inch heavy-weight drawing paper

1. Choose a color that reflects how you're feeling today.

2. Draw a circle with that color.

3. In that circle, use lines and shapes to draw an image or images to identify how you're feeling today.

4. Name your art.

25. Finding Shorty

The summer has broken out in the small village of Salbruck. Libby and her friends have long been waiting for the big heat wave to finally be able to bathe again at the Lasse quarry. Already in the morning the air smells of summer. Libby is on his way to Poppel to pick him up at school. Alex is coming too. At the corner of the Gaus-Alle Libby makes as usual a larger arc around the house of the old Bellbi. Old Bellbi has been living there for ages. At least he looks like this. Somehow the old man has something scary with all the wrinkles on his face and bony hands.

Libby and her friends once danced on Bellbi's property. Of course he caught her. Old Bellbi just gets it all. As if he had his eyes and ears everywhere. He chased the children from his property with his cane in hand. Since then, they have avoided the house.

Libby is driving past the house. Usually it is the same picture every morning. The old Bellbi stands on his lawn bleating and complaining to the neighbor, because his dog has allegedly done his business there again. The neighbor does not answer anymore. He takes his daughter to the car and pretends he does not hear Bellbi. That makes old Bellbi so mad that he gets louder.

The three friends have also seen how the old Bellbi complained loudly to his neighbor, because the dog had barked all night. He barely had an eye - heard the old man yelling. Whereby the dog of the Knigges really likes to bark at night. At least that's what Libby's mom says. She often protects old Bellbi and always tells how friendly he used to be when Mrs. Bellbi was still alive.

But today, nothing is to be seen or heard of old Bellbi. Also Mr. Knigge is not - as usual - in the driveway. Libby stops for a moment and scratches his head thoughtfully. "That's funny," she thinks. "Did something happen to old Bellbi?" She would like to check. But he does not dare and then he continues.

After a few minutes, Libby arrives at Poppel. Of course, Poppel is not his real name. Actually his name is Holger. But because he is a bit more stable, it looks kind of funny when he runs. At some point, Alex said: "Look, Holger comes running hoppeldipoppel." Alex and Libby had to laugh so hard that they called Holger from then only Poppel. By now he's so used to hearing Holger.

Alex is coming too. "Hey Alex - almost at the same time - what?" Libby shouts to Alex. Alex grins: "Oh, Libby, did not even see you - yes, funny." Then the front door flies open and Poppel trumpets: "Well send her thick - everything in step?" That's Poppel's typical way. Always the big mouth in front path.

Libby shakes his head: "I think you'll never change Poppel!" Poppel beams over his ears: "But never my dear Libby - you sweetie!" He says and shakes Libby's hand. Libby has to laugh. But then she gets serious: "Hey guys, you know what I've been watching today? Old Bellbi was not complaining. "Poppel is closing his bike lock:" Oh, well, did he swallow himself or what? "Libby shakes his head:" No, seriously. He was not there. And Knigge was not in the driveway. I was thinking about looking to see if something had happened to the old Bellbi. "

Alex thinks: "Funny it is." But Poppel interferes immediately: "Nah no people, you can forget that right away. You probably do not remember how the old Zausel chased us off the grounds with a fat club. You can eat that nice. The thick one always gets it first! I can not get ten more horses! "Libby rolls her eyes:" Oh Poppel, you always have to overdo everything! That was a walking stick and not a club! "

Poppel waves down: "I do not care what you tell Libby. In my story that was a fat stick and I'll stick with it. "Alex shakes his head but then says," Either way, Poppel is right Libby. That brings nothing but trouble. In addition, we are slowly getting late. We should really go to school. If I'm late again, my dad turns right on the bike. "Libby nods and the three go.

The school day passes quickly and Libby does not mention the topic with the old Bellbi anymore. In the afternoon, the three friends drive to the Lasse quarry to test the water for temperature. Libby keeps his foot in the water and immediately winced. "Brrrr, is that still cold! The lake has probably not noticed the summer is. "Alex and Poppel laugh. Then Alex says, "We'll keep those few days off now. In addition, soon holidays. "Poppel nods:" Right! I am already counting the days. We have another week until the summer holidays. Then it will finally be donated again! Stop schoolwork and stuff! "

The next morning Libby drives her track as usual to pick up Poppel. But there is no sign of old Bellbi. Shortly before Poppel's house she sees Mr. Knigge, who is putting a leaflet on the fence. Libby stops to look at it. On the leaflet is a missing message for the dog of the Knigges. "That makes sense," she thinks. "If the King's dog ran away, then old Bellbi has no reason to complain."

Mr. Knigge sees Libby and approaches: "Hello Libby, Shorty disappeared the night before last night. While I have no hope that anyone will get in touch with the leaflets, if you see something, please call - yes? "Libby nods." Of course, Mr. Knigge, I'll do that for sure. "Libby had a summer last summer Watch out for the dog of the Knigges and has since gone to Shorty Gassi or played the dog sitter on weekends. Shorty has since become pretty fond of Libby.

Libby just wants to continue driving, as she stops again: "Mr. Knigge? It's a nice shock to me that Shorty ran away. I really hope they find him again. "Mr. Knigge turns around:" Many thanks Libby, but all the doors and windows were locked. I do not think he ran away. "Libby looks dumbfounded," Is that someone's kidnapping Shorty? "Mr. Knigge nods," It looks like it. "Libby is not sure what to answer:" That's it Yes unbelievable! Then I keep my eyes open in any case, "she says and goes on.

On the way to school Libby tells Alex and Poppel the whole story. Alex is horrified: "That's a strong piece! A dog hijack here in Salbruck? That's probably the most exciting thing that ever happened here, is it? "Libby agrees:" I agree. Do you think the old Bellbi has anything to do with it? "Alex shakes his head." Oh shit. He is at least 100 years old - how should he have anything to do with it? "Libby continues:" Just think, the old Bellbi has the biggest motive. He is constantly complaining about the dog. "

Poppel intervenes - somewhat out of breath from cycling - "Libby is right!" Poppel gasps: "I trust the old man too." Now he interrupts: "Hey guys, maybe we can stop, if we talk? I get gasp breathing! "The three friends stop and Poppel is breathing hard. "Ok, suppose old Bellbi had the faxes thick. What could be more appropriate than to make the dog disappear? "

Alex is not quite sure: "But how should he have done that?" Libby is very excited: "That's exactly what it needs to find out! We'll convict old Bellbi! "Poppel shakes his head." No, no, no, yesterday I did not make my point clear enough. I do not want to have anything to do with old Bellbi! "Libby looks at Poppel." Poppel, do not you want to pay the old man back? "

Poppel thinks for a moment. Then he answers: "Damn, yes, that sounds good. Then I play stick out of the bag! "Libby looks over to Alex:" Are you there too? "Alex hesitates, but then he agrees and extends his hand:" Oh, hell. Then the three musketeers are reunited. "Libby and Poppel put their hands on Alex's hand. Then all three cheer at the same time: "One for all and all for one!"

In the afternoon, the three hide in the bushes on the opposite side of the Bellbi House. Poppel has his binoculars for shading. "I did not know that so many people come by every day!" Says Alex. Libby says, "And we're not the only ones who suspect Bellbi," she says. "Did you see how they all shake their heads when they pass Bellbi's house?" Suddenly Poppel makes a cramped sound: "Ooh, have you seen that? Lisa's mother just passed by and trampled on the flowerbed of old Bellbi. "

Alex reaches for the binoculars: "Show me! Fact, not a lie. Everything flat! Libby look. "Alex holds out the binoculars to Libby, but Libby does not take it. "What's going on?" Asks Alex. Libby looks thoughtful: "What if we do wrong to old Bellbi? If he was not?

Everyone seems to think that old Bellbi has kidnapped the dog or worse. "

Poppel babbles immediately: "Are you kidding me Libby? And if that was the old stick vibrator! Anyone who goes after children, but before all animals has no respect! "Alex holds Poppel on the shoulder:" Wait Poppel. Libby is right! On television it is always - in doubt for the defendant. "Then he turns to Libby:" Listen to Libby. Even if he was not, we are his best chance of enlightenment. We're only here to find out the truth. "

Poppel puffs himself up: "To find out the truth? I think it hacks. I'm here to mop up the old Bellbi. "Alex shuts Poppel's mouth, still trying to keep talking," Hmmmmmmmmmmmmmm. "Poppel frees his mouth," That's good. I understood. We're here to play Samaritan, for an old guy who did not deserve this. Alright Libby. I'm still here! After all, there is a chance that he is guilty and then I want to be there when the handcuffs click. "Alex looks at Libby:" All right Libby? "Libby nods:" All right! Let's find out the truth. "

Slowly dawn breaks and old Bellbi was not even visible. "Good that we told our parents that we're having an overnight party with you - Poppel," says Alex. "Class idea?" Replies Poppel. But Libby is not that enthusiastic: "Well, I did not think it was great to fool my parents." Poppel shakes his head: "Nonsense with sauce! We all spend the night together. What was lying there? "Alex looks at Libby:" Well, you have to admit, somehow that makes sense. "Libby nods:" That really makes sense. "Poppel interrupts the whole thing:" Pssst, well, rest now! It is dark! The mission begins. "

The three friends sneak across the street to the old Bellbi's fence. "Down Alex!" Hisses Poppel. "I can not go down. I'm just taller than you! "Libby intervenes:" Rest now you two or we'll fly up! "They sneak along the fence to the backyard. "Look," says Poppel. "An open window. Here we go. Avoid skid marks in underpants! "Then Poppel flits to the open window. "What's he doing there?" Asks Libby. "Was that the plan?" Alex shakes his head. "We did not have a plan. Come on! "Then he starts running too.

Poppel hangs on the window sill with his legs wriggling. "Now push one," he whispers. Alex tries to get his legs under control: "Shit, not so loud and stop fidgeting!" Suddenly Poppel stops fidgeting and stays still. "Did you hear that too?" He asks. Alex answers, "What's the matter?" And turns to Libby. Libby nods: "Yeah, I heard it too." Alex gets restless: "Yeah what? Is old Bellbi coming with a truncheon? "" No! "Whispers Poppel. "Then I would be over all mountains!" Libby looks around: "That was a soft barking. Well, as suppressed as a woof. But that did not come from here. "

Alex pulls Poppel out of the window. "Boy, put that on my stomach." Poppel complains. "I really have to lose weight! But the noise came, I think, from across. "Alex is surprised:" Of the Knigges? Did the Shorty find again? "Libby pats Alex's forehead with the palm of his hand." Man, think about it, Alex! What would be the best way to show that the old Bellbi is not quite ticking anymore? The Knigges just pretended that Shorty was kidnapped. "Alex shakes his head," I do not believe it! "Libby nods to Alex," That's exactly what it is. Who would suspect that? Even I would not trust Mr. Knigge. "

Poppel is visibly disappointed: "Shit, and I wanted to wipe the old dry bean one. That will be nothing. But how can we prove now that the Knigges have only faked the kidnapping? "The three friends think. Then Alex says: "Helps nothing. Then we have to go in for the Knigges and convince ourselves. "Libby skin Alex again on the forehead:" Super idea Intelligence bolt. And then they put it down to kidnap and bring back Shorty. "Poppel has to stop laughing:" She's right, you're not the brightest chandelier in the chandelier, Alex. "Alex glares at Poppel:" Ha ha, very funny dickers. "Libby walks between the two:" Now stop! I have an idea."

After half an hour you hear police sirens approaching the House of the Knigges. Two patrol cars and a police car stop in front of the house. A handful of police rush to the door. Just as they want to break open the door, it swings open and Mr. Knigge stands in the doorway. "What's happening? So much police for a dog hijacking? Did you find Shorty? "

The policeman looks surprised: "We have received a call from her daughter that the abductor is now in the house." Mr. Knigge shakes his head: "That's nonsense. My daughter is sleeping soundly. "But the policeman persists:" Mr. Knigge, please step aside. We need to be sure. "Mr. Knigge stops in the doorway," And I tell them - they will not search my house. "Two police officers take Mr. Knigge aside and the rest of the forces search the house.

When the police come out, one of the officers wears Shorty in his arms. "Um, Mr. Knigge, will you explain that to me please?" Mr. Knigge reaches for the dog: "Yes, I did not mention that, Shorty was brought back. Thank God! "The policeman takes a step back and keeps the dog in his arms. "When we arrived, they asked if we had found their dog. In addition, her daughter actually slept and can not have called accordingly to the police. We must now clarify this situation. "

At this moment, Libby, Alex and Poppel are brought to the front door of the Knigge by one of the other policemen. "And who are you?" Asks the policeman with the dog in his arms. Libby tells the whole story and apologizes for lying on the phone. The policeman bends down to her. "All right, little lady. As Chief Inspector, I tell you, you've done just the thing - calling the police. It would have been better, however, to tell the truth. "Then the commissioner smiles:" On the other side, not everything was lying. "And looks at Mr. Knigge. "The dog hijacker was really in the house. Is that right, Herr Knigge? "

When the Commissioner addresses Mr. Knigge directly, it breaks out of him: "I only did that because I was desperate. Every day the bleating of old Bellbi. I could not stand it anymore. "The commissioner nods:" All right, Mr. Knigge, but there are definitely other ways. Please accompany us to the guard now. "Two policemen bring Mr. Knigge to the patrol car.

Then the inspector looks again at Libby, Alex and Poppel: "And now we bring you three home better." Poppel shakes his head and waves: "No, not necessary. I'll go alone. See you guys! "But the commissioner stops him:" Do not worry my boy. You are almost heroes. Your parents will be proud of you. But we still need your statements and that's best done together with your parents. And after that you should go to bed too, right? "

Poppel shines all over his face: "Heroes? Yes, I want to be a hero. I always knew that. It's time for my parents to find out about it and the school and the city ... "While Poppel is still chattering, the three are taken to the patrol car.

Libby is still stunned that Mr. Knigge himself was the dog hijacker: "It's hard to believe that Mr. Knigge was himself. I can not believe it, "says Libby. Poppel grins and pulls Alex up. "Yes, Alex, tell me that as the brightest light in the chandelier - can you believe it?" He sneers. Alex snappily answers: "Not everyone can be such a great hero as you hoppeldipoppel!" And everyone laughs.

24. The Sleep Rainbow

Take in a big, deep breath. Focus on the air as it goes into your body and hold it there. Then, exhale slowly and deeply. Do this again, and as you do it, imagine that your lungs are great, big balloons. Fill them up as much as you possibly can without popping them, and then hold the air within them for the count of five. Five... Four... Three... Two... One... Now, gently exhale your breath through your mouth, blowing it through your lips as if you were blowing out a candle, focusing carefully not to blow it too quickly.

Breathe again... And again...

Now, find your comfortable position in bed. Make sure that it is exactly right, and try not to move as we continue with the meditation. When you are ready, you can move on.

Breathe again and again... Let the breath slowly fill your lungs and be exhaled. With this next breath, as you breathe in, imagine that all of the tension from the day is going into your lungs. Let all of that tension that you were holding up within you go in, just as the carbon dioxide transfers into your breath. Hold it there just long enough to let all of the tension build up... And then, let it go once more. As you exhale, imagine that the tension in your body is blowing away. Feel how your body becomes free of its weight.

You notice that your body is feeling very calm and relaxed now at this point. It is feeling heavier than ever, and you are not sure if you would be able to move it, even if you wanted to. You feel each and every muscle releasing, allowing you to sink deeper and deeper into your bed. Even your jaw feels relaxed, and all tension has melted away from your body. As we continue through this meditation, imagine that your body is growing calmer and calmer. You will feel it release out tension that you did not know that you even had, and that is a good thing—it shows that your relaxation is working.

Now, close your eyes if they are not already closed. Take another breath. If you feel any more tension in your body, let it out with your exhale.

Focus inwardly as much as you can. Focus on the feeling of air in your chest and then let go of that focus entirely. Your mind is just as relaxed as your body now, and you are not thinking about anything else; you are simply listening to the words of this meditation.

In your mind's eye, you see something in front of you—it is a rainbow, arching down from the sky and touching the ground, right in front of you. You can see the entire rainbow and the whole spectrum of colors, from red to violet, all right in front of you. You reach out to touch the rainbow, and you realize that each and every color feels different, and your own breaths match the colors that you are touching. As you put your hand in the middle of all of the colors, your breath becomes visible to you as you continue to breathe; in your mind, you can see your breath as a rainbow cloud that you slowly and gently exhale, as it wafts up into the air around you.

First, you touch the red of the rainbow, and immediately, your breath shifts. With your next exhale, you can see the red leaving your lungs. As you breathe in, imagine that all of your anger from the day is filling up your lungs. As your hand is in the red, your lungs begin to gather up all of that anger that is still pent up within you. Imagine your frustrations from the day as you continue to absorb them, and then let them go. Every time you breathe out while your hand is in the red color, you breathe out more and more of your anger. Keep doing this until you have erased all of your anger from the day. You are releasing it back out into the world, leaving space in your heart for what is to come next.

With all of your anger out of your heart, you reach over to orange. The orange in the rainbow feels different from the red; it feels like you are touching something that is cold. This is the color of all of your anxieties from the day, and you are going to release them as the orange of the rainbow washes over you. Keep your hand on the orange and slowly, but surely, imagine that all of your anxiety from the day is entering your lungs to be exhaled. As you do this, little by little, you relieve that anxiety from yourself. With every breath that you take in, your lungs expand and fill with that anxiety. Then, you are able to breathe it out. You can see the clouds of orange emanating from your mouth as you exhale.

Now, your hand moves over toward yellow, and in touching yellow, you feel the fatigue of your day, all of that exhaustion and drain that you have built up over the course of getting through your general day, fade away. You can feel it all building within you, just like you could feel that anger and that anxiety. You will it all to go toward your lungs, one by one, so you can expel it out into the world. You cannot make space for the wonderful feelings that will help you to go to sleep if you are too filled up with those negative feelings, so you must let them all out, one by one, breath by breath.

With all of that negativity out of your body, you notice that you feel much more relaxed. Your body continues to sink into your bed and you begin to feel very heavy as you do so. You are beginning to feel the inkling of tiredness at the edge of your consciousness, but you know that it is not yet time to go to sleep. You are not empty right now, after you have released all of that negative energy; rather, you are filled with endless potential. You have the potential to become anything at all right now as you sit there, looking at the rainbow in front of you. The red, the orange, and the yellow streaks on the rainbow all seem to have brightened up; the rainbow has taken that negativity away from you, leaving space for everything else that can follow.

Take in a deep breath again, and another exhale. Now, will yourself, in your mind, to move your hand out toward the green stripe on the rainbow in front of you. You reach into the green, and you are greeted with the feeling of a friend's hand on your own; it is that same comfortable, familiar warmth that you feel when you get to spend time with your best friend. It is that same sense of amicability, that sense of being able to interact with ease. It is that ability to just look at someone else and know that, at the end of the day, they are on your side. It is the feeling of a friend's embrace and the platonic love that you get from all around you.

Now, this is not something that you want to leave behind; this is a gift from the rainbow to you as you prepare to go to sleep. This is what the rainbow has prepared just for you to help you begin to relax once and for all. As you touch this color, you notice, your breath does not change at all when you breathe out. But, when you breathe in, you can see the green from the rainbow coming toward the air that you are breathing. You can feel the warmth of your friendships emanating into your lungs, and you can feel that warmth dissipating over the rest of your body as well. You can sense the love that your friends have for you within your body, reminding you of a very important point: You are loved. Your friends love you.

When you have absorbed all of the feeling of love that you can from your friends, it is time to move to the next color in the rainbow: Blue. Many people think that blue is a sad color, but it is not, at all. Blue is dependable, like the sky; you know that it will always be there. Blue is confident, like the sea; it can rise to any occasion. It is trustworthy; it is that look of admiration that a child give to you when you tell them that you achieved something that they could only dream of, even if that something was something entirely ordinary in the adult world, such as cooking something from scratch. Blue is the feeling of wisdom, of knowing when to act and when to not. It is the color of imagination and inspiration.

As you hold your hand into the blue of the rainbow, you feel trust, both in yourself and in those that you know are trustworthy in your life. With every breath, you are filled with that necessary self-confidence that you need to succeed. The blue will remind you to feel like you are dependable; you are reliable and trustworthy. You can trust your judgment any time that you have it; there is no reason that you have to balk away from it. You breathe in the blue and with it, you breathe in that gentle, but stable trust that you need for yourself.

When you have finished inhaling in the blue trust, you move over to indigo. As you touch the color, you feel your heart swell up. You feel the feeling of a hug from a loved one; that sensation of being truly cherished and valued beyond that of a platonic friend. It is that feeling that you are dear to someone's heart, that feeling of hugging them tightly and closely, and as you breathe in the indigo from the rainbow, you feel cherished. You are reminded that you are adored by people in this world, whether that is by a spouse or a romantic partner, or by your parents, your children, or other family, or even your best friends. Someone in this world, or maybe even many people in this world, cherish you deeply and you revel in that.

Finally, as your hand is guided into the violet of the rainbow, you realize something. You are overcome by a sensation of deep, heavy relaxation. You can feel the hand of a true friend on your shoulder. You can feel the steadfast confidence and trust in yourself in your heart, and you can feel the feeling of being cherished throughout your whole body. All of that comes together, creating the violet waves of exhaustion that wash over you. With each and every deep breath that you take, you feel yourself growing calmer and calmer. You find yourself being bathed in that violet light from the rainbow, even after you move your hand. With every breath that you take, remember that the violet calmness is washing over you. Continue to breathe deeply until you finally drift asleep, bathed in violet with green on your hand, blue in your heart and indigo wrapped around your body.

25. The Famous Writer

Norman Alderman was a single man of the age of 48. Each and every new day, he worried more about being single. It was 2012, and all of his friends, by this time, had children, and some of them even had grandchildren. But then he thought, "I guess I shouldn't worry about that because we are all different now, aren't we?" Norman was taken to standing in front of the mirror, seeing himself as a playwright or famous novelist receiving a Pulitzer for his magnificent work. What Norman saw in that mirror was Charlton Heston. What the mirror showed was Woody Allen. He did have one redeeming feature, though; he was smart. At least he thought he was smart. "Aren't all people like me smart?" he mused.

Norman was a writer. He thought he had what it takes. Actually, that's not true. He was trained to be an accountant. He had worked in that field for six years and saw himself as a tiny little man at a tiny little desk in a huge office full of tiny little people. He did not like that view, so every day, he went home and meditated. While in his meditative state, he tried to make himself wake up a famous and successful writer, but every time he pulled out of it, he was still a silly little ineffectual, Jewish man. "Well, at least I'm good at meditating," he thought.

Norman was a persistent man, although, at times, he wondered what he should do with his free time, should he quit writing and do something else. "No," he thought, "that would be giving up, and I'm not a quitter. I'm not," he repeated to himself in his mind. "I write, therefore I am a writer!" he exclaimed to himself. "Who am I talking to?" he asked, hoping nobody else ever heard these musings should they think of him as wonky. So, Norman wrote. He wrote poems, short stories, and articles. He had files of pieces that he had written. All of them good, but all of them good enough. "If I can just get that winning piece, that one literary achievement." He muttered. "If I could just do it?" Each evening when he went to bed, he saw himself as a great writer; he just knew he had it in him. If it would only come out

It was Friday afternoon, and he had just got home from work at his accounting job. He thought about calling his friend, who was also an accountant and who also wore horn-rimmed glasses, like him, but she wasn't a writer. She was a real accountant. In fact, she was the boss's number one bean counter. "I think the boss is a little like me, a little lonely. That's probably why he likes her?" he questioned in his mind.

One thing that you should know about Norman is that he is eccentric. He loved his computer and owned an old tower that he just kept fixing. He also owned a laptop, but he wrote on neither of these machines. He had inherited an old Remington Rand from a family estate, and he felt that the machine gave his writing work character. In fact, he felt that the old machine gave him character.

That night, Norman had an idea. He scrambled over to his typewriter, dropped into his seat, and placed a brand-new blank sheet of typing paper in the machine. "Let's see now," he said. "What can we call this piece? I know," he said excitedly. "We'll call it the writer!" He placed his palms facing outwards, interlocked his fingers, and pushed out cracking all of his knuckles at the same time. Then he placed his hands in the writing position on the typewriter keyboard. When he began to type, something magical happened. It was as though his fingers were doing the thinking.

they flew over the keys getting far ahead of his mind. How can this be, he asked?

He looked up at the clock. "Wait a minute now?" He said. "I know that the clock is at twenty after four because I just looked at it a minute ago. Now it says 6:30? This is amazing," he said, "but it can't be?" he thought. "I just work for 2 hours? There must be some missing time somewhere." But when he looked down at what he had written, he skidded his chair back wildly and tore the paper from the typewriter. "Did I write that? I wrote this! I did it! I do have the touch!" Then, realizing that the piece was only just begun, he replaced the paper in return and sat down again to continue. A small amount of drool emanated from the right corner of his lips. He didn't notice this. He was so deeply involved in what was happening. He felt a strange power overtaking him. At first, he thought, "Well, this is not right?" but then he said, "The heck with that! This is me! This is me doing what I do best. I am the writer!"

Norman typed and typed! He typed on that old Remington until midnight and then typed some more. He wasn't even looking over the script that he was writing; he did no "on the fly" proofreading at all. This wasn't like him. He usually took more time staring at what he had written than doing the writing itself, and this gave him thought. At 2 AM, he stopped. His writing was scaring him.

At one point, before sliding the chair back from the desk, he thought, "this is just wrong! I like being in control of me." But when he read over what his crazed fingers had written, all that went out the window. Why he had written about himself, or at least that's what he thought at first. But when he got into the piece, he noticed that the man's name was Chad. "That's not me?" he said to himself. Then he read the entire piece and began to write more.

Chad was an attorney but had never won a single case. The state put him in charge of handling the defendants who couldn't afford to hire their own attorney. He was a "Court Appointed Lawyer" and a loser. The problem was that his heart wasn't into it. He wondered how he could have picked the wrong career. He wanted to be a writer, so every night, he wrote. "The small and fruitless man sat down at his computer and began to write. He wrote and wrote until his fingers were tired, and his brain was on fire. The story took the form of a woman by the name of Edna, who was a writer, and had no confidence, but kept on writing day after day anyway, and did finally produce something she liked.

At first, Edna thought that she was writing about herself, but then she noticed that she had typed a name. The character was called Joyce, and Joyce was a winner. She entered contests and won them. She didn't know why, and she had no plan that could possibly be called a system, she just won. Why just last week, Edna wrote, Joyce had won a brand-new car. It was just a little front-wheel-drive Ford with a tiny little engine that sat sideways in the front. Joyce was happy with it though although Edna wrote, she was worried that she would have to pay some sort of tax on her new car value when April rolled around again. The following month, Edna wrote about Joyce again and decided that Joyce, would enter the Readers Digest Sweepstakes. Of course, she won the big prize, which was no surprise to Edna as that was all in the script as the saying goes. Edna wrote that Joyce was overjoyed but not surprised and she won half a million dollars and just put it in the bank, and kept on living the same way as if nothing great had happened.

Norman loved his coffee, and sometimes on the weekends, he would take his laptop and sit in the local coffee shop drinking coffee and writing. It was a Saturday morning, and he decided that this would be one of those days. He packed up his trusty old laptop and headed out. When Norman arrived at the coffee shop, he realized it was still very early, and the place was nearly empty. "Where shall we sit this morning?" he asked himself. "Ah, the table in the back, that's where we'll park it." He sat down and plugged in his computer and then went up and ordered his coffee and a pastry.

He cracked his knuckles the way he always did before he started to write, and then returned to his work in progress. The story about the writer named Chad. He wrote for a long time and didn't notice that the shop had become very crowded. A woman had taken the seat across the table from him but way down at the other end, and then a young man came in the shop with his laptop and looked around. He noticed the empty seat next to Norman and walked over. "Do you mind if I sit here and work?" he asked Norman. "Be my guest," Norman said without looking up from his screen. He heard the man shuffling around and plugging in his machine but paid no heed. He was a writer, and he must write.

Then Chad suddenly sneezed, and Norman said, "Gesundheit." "Thank you," the young man said. "Are you a writer?" the man asked and then, "I'm sorry, may I introduce myself, my name is Chad." The man said. Norman's head jerked up in surprise. After typing the name Chad over and over for the last month or so, he was shocked to suddenly meet a man with the same name. He noticed that Chad was holding his hand out and waiting to shake Norman's hand in their meeting. "Uh, oh sorry," Norman said, "I'm Norman, and yes, I am a writer." "Me too," Chad told him.

"Now this was starting to be very freaky, Norman thought. Could there be this kind of coincidence?" he wondered. They both returned to their respective laptops, and another half hour passed. Then Chad got up and went into the restroom and left his computer open. Norman thought, "Oh no, you don't? That would be very disrespectful. After all, you wouldn't want anyone looking over your shoulder trying to see what you were writing." But he couldn't control his curiosity, and he knew that was a weakness. He looked. He saw the word Edna and almost jumped out of his skin. He looked again and noticed that in Chad's story, Edna was also a writer. "This just can't be!" he thought in a panic.

Exercise

Prioritize items on the list. By indicating which items are high priority, you can be sure to do those ones first and can relax about not getting to the lower-priority items right away.

Ready to make your own to-do list using these principles? You can use the template below to write down activities you need to complete, including their due date. Then give each task a priority level (e.g., low/medium/high, or 0–10). Finally, schedule a time in your calendar to complete each activity.

26. On a Hot Air Balloon

You feel the excitement and nervousness in your restless body as you approach the gigantic balloon. Climbing into the wicker basket, you feel your heart flutter, and your stomach does a small flip.

You can smell the propane and hear the burning flame ready to power this balloon into the air. Holding onto the edge of the basket, you wait for your secure ascent into the air. Feeling the smooth wood beneath your hand, the drift of the slightest amount of heat from the balloon, the distant smell of a salty ocean. As the basket starts to rise, you feel how tense and achy your muscles are. You concentrate on grounding yourself as your body is being lifted to unknown heights.

Digging your toes down into the floor of the basket. Feeling your strong, sturdy ankles supporting you letting you know they won't waver; they will keep you steady.

Your legs feel alive as the muscles reflectively tense and relax as you ground yourself. As you rise even higher, you feel a shift in your body.

The fear of the flight is leaving you; instead, you feel an uplifting grace and peaceful presence.

Your body doesn't feel as heavy as it did moments ago.

The almost weightlessness you experience settles you. As you look around at the beautiful scenery, you continue to stabilize your body. You are relaxing your aching back, allowing the curves to blend into themselves.

Your stomach is settling down as you focus your thoughts on your breathing. Breathing in and expanding your lungs, delivering oxygen to your body, and breathing out, allowing your muscles to relax and await their next oxygen delivery.

As you breathe in and out slowly, you can relax your shoulders, neck, and finally, your mind.

As you continue relaxing and breathing, you can focus on the land growing smaller beneath you. Like the troubles, you leave behind when you sleep.

The balloon drifts peacefully, and you can see the ocean now. The water is deep blue, the beach over-crowded, and people are eager to find the blissful relaxation you're already experiencing.

The red and white umbrellas line the crowded beach, people lying on their towels on the warm sand. You're above the beach now, and people point, and you can hear them hoot and holler as you soar above.

Hearing the ocean lull beneath the sound of the crowd. You wave hello with a warm smile, thankful you can easily slip away from this crowded area and into your cocoon of happiness and warmth.

The balloon drifts further from the crowd and noises. The ocean is shrinking and becoming distant. You can no longer smell or hear the bustle that was on the ocean shore. Now, your mind is welcoming the quiet uninhabited lands you are approaching. Your nose is eager for the clean, crisp scents of the fields beneath you.

Seeing many colors of wildflowers blur together as you soar above. Like a bird in a lengthy flight for winter, you take in all your surroundings.

Relaxing, breathing, just being.

You are traveling away for your long, peaceful rest. Stepping away from the cold harshness that can sometimes be a reality, and traveling to the warm, sunny peace deep inside your mind. Below you see a laundry line and a small farmhouse; seeing the clothing dance on the line as you gently pass by as if now, they are waving to you as you waved to the beachgoers. The land turns from flat and uninhabited to small rolling hills with the occasional house.

You see, the town grows as you travel towards the center, roads, houses, and more businesses.

As the path of your life, you start fresh, not knowing many things, being able to see and know everything around you like the small farmhouse.

As you age, the roads you travel become familiar, but longer, more complicated, twists and turns, connecting to other roads. The houses keep popping up as you meet new people. The businesses are opportunities that you may latch onto or let them pass by, whichever is right for you at that time in your life. The connections throughout this town or city, working like your mind, often do. You are growing together, supporting a singular body.

You pass over neighborhoods, seeing the quiet towns below. Friendly neighbors have cookouts and children playing kickball together.

The towns pass by so quickly, and it reminds you of how quickly time can seem to pass. Your mind tries to distract you, remind you of the things you need to accomplish.

The things you need to worry about. It's time to quiet those thoughts.

You are creating your wind as you soar through the sky, whisper your concerns to the wind.

Let them travel through the air, fall to the ground. You can pick them up at another time. Whisper the thoughts of what you need to do tomorrow. Whisper the thoughts of what you should be worrying about.

Whisper anything that is on your mind. Watch the words leave your mouth, drift through your wind, fall to the ground. The words are jumbling together as they spiral to the ground. Falling and falling until you can no longer see them.

Those thoughts are gone now; you have freed your mind and have total control over your body.

Breathing in allowing your body to soak in the peace with a clear mind. Breathing out, feeling your body sigh with relief.

The hot air balloon is now traveling over the forest. The tops of the trees are green and lush. You feel like a cloud floating above the trees. The coverage dense in some areas, shielding you from the world below. While in other areas, it thins out, allowing you to peek at the wonderful mother nature has set before you.

A group of birds' flocks beside you can hear them calling out to each other at the curiosity you are presenting to them in this huge balloon.

How odd it must be for them. You look up and are again amazed at how a little bit of heat and this huge material are allowing you to soar with birds. The rainbow color panels seem to glow as the sun shines down through them.

The red panel was making you think of love and warmth. The orange panel was reminding you of tropical colors on an island, the flowers, the clothes, the fruits, and the peaceful setting sun.

The yellow panel reminds you of pure happiness and joy, like a full warm sun, or the tart bite of a lemon.

The green panel is showing the reflection of life; of mother nature as it surrounds you...the green of the trees, the grass, the fields below.

The blue panel, reflecting on the open, clear skies.

Open like your mind, absorbing the welcoming warmth of the other colors.

The purple panel reflects its vibrant color that can be rarer than the others and is often a sign of nobility—reflecting the rare peace and calm of complete bliss, reflecting this journey in this hot air balloon.

The forest is thinning out, and you can see a beach in the distance. As you approach it, you find yourself approaching a barely sandy and more rocky shore, the water angrily lapping at the shoreline.

While not friendly for a relaxing day at the beach, the sounds of the crashing waves reflect that of your beating heart. It's as if you can feel those waves beating against the rocks from deep within your soul.

You feel the blood pumping through your body, then beating through your heart. The waves are rolling in and out like your breath and working together to create a beautiful rhythm that is essential for your life.

The ocean's sounds start to drift off until you only feel your heart, mirroring what you know the ocean is doing even in your absence.

You approach an open field; you know your journey must be near its end. As the balloon starts to descend, you feel yourself falling slightly more horizontal.

I was peacefully drifting into the proper place of relaxation.

Your body shifts, finding the most comforting position as you feel the weight returning to your body.

The heaviness is weighing your body down until it feels impossible to do nothing but let it pull you down. Relax into the weight.

Feel your body sinking into the warmth of the descent. Allow your tired legs to rest, pulling the rest of your body down with them. Breath in and out slowly as you drift down into peace, lying your head back and feeling gravity welcome you home.

The warmth of the balloon envelopes you as you caress the ground. The balloon is at rest. Lie here as long as you like. Rest, breathe in the field around you.

What does this field look like up closely?

Are its fragrant flowers?

Warm and mellow wheat?

Close your eyes and rest for a moment.

Allow your body to sink in and enjoy this complete relaxation this trip has brought you. Reflect on the sights that you have seen, and only one thing stirs you from your revelry… The pilot asks you, "Do you want to go up again?"

www.ingramcontent.com/pod-product-compliance
Lightning Source LLC
Chambersburg PA
CBHW052203090526
44583CB00015BA/1259